UNLOCKING WELLNESS: NATURAL HERBAL REMEDIES FOR DISEASES

EMPOWER YOURSELF WITH HERBAL KNOWLEDGE, REDUCE UNWANTED SIDE EFFECTS NATURALLY, ACHIEVE LONG-TERM WELLNESS WITH HERBAL MEDICINE

RAMI ARCHER

DRW
PUBLISHING VENTURES

TABLE OF CONTENTS

INTRODUCTION

Herbal remedy practice is a thread that weaves through the tapestry of human history, connecting cultures and civilizations across the globe—and across time. From the Amazonian rainforests to ancient Egyptian and Chinese cultures, to the medieval apothecaries of Europe, to the indigenous tribes of the Americas, knowledge of plant-based healing has long been a cornerstone of human health and wellness.

Yet, as our world veers towards a future dominated by technological advancements and synthetic medicines, the profound relevance of these ancient practices has never been more applicable. Contemporary societies are grappling with the limitations of modern medicine —especially in the face of illnesses that resist modern treatments— and our most needed answers may well lie in the heart of this ancient wisdom. Deeply rooted in the earth's rhythm and the cycles of nature, it offers a reminder of our past and a beacon for our future at a critical time.

I'm Rami Archer, and I'm pleased to guide you on this enlightening journey. My early passion for holistic health ignited in the lush greenery of my grandmother's garden, a breathtaking place where plants served as flora and friends, each holding stories and secrets of their own. This connection with nature led me to explore the depths of herbal remedies, leading to a profound realization: *nature holds the key to our health and wellness*. With a heart full of this ancient wisdom and a spirit driven by a mission to empower, I've dedicated myself to sharing and spreading herbal medicine's healing power. My aim now? I want to empower *you* with this knowledge for self-care, allowing you to take control of your health and wellness journey.

Herbal healing is a call to embrace the balance between tradition and innovation—between yesterday and tomorrow. Its great potential underscores the importance of preserving our natural heritage and learning from the earth. As we collectively navigate the challenges of the 21st century, the ancient wisdom and practices serve as an enduring bedrock testament to nature's power to heal, sustain, and teach. They inspire and guide us toward a future where health and healing are rooted in the most profound respect for our natural world.

Modern society's resurging interest in natural health solutions speaks volumes about herbal remedies' efficacy, affordability, and minimal side effects. This book draws on statistics and influential new studies and stands at the intersection of tradition and science, offering a trusted guide to nature's pharmacy. This book aims to accompany you as you explore the nurturing embrace of nature, turning to the surrounding green world for healing, understanding, and a sense of community. By engaging with these pages, you're not just reading; you're stepping into a realm where every leaf and root has a story, each with the potential to change your life.

Our journey together will demystify the world of herbal remedies, bringing ancient wisdom into the light of the modern day. We'll dispel myths that have long clouded insight into the true efficacy of herbal medicine, illuminating a path as enriching as it is empowering. This book covers practical applications in our daily lives today, serving as a roadmap to personalizing your health and wellness journey with nature's bounty.

I understand that stepping away from conventional medicine can be challenging and daunting for many. You may have faced skepticism, fears, or disappointments in the past—or you may still be facing them today. Here, I promise you a discovery of real, actionable solutions. Esteemed figures in the holistic health and herbal medicine community have lent their voices to support this work, affirming its value and reliability.

You can expect to find knowledge, understanding, and a new perspective on health and wellness in these pages. I offer unique and actionable insights about creating your own herbal remedies and integrating herbal practices into your daily life. I encourage you to approach this information with an open heart and a curious mind. Let this be the beginning of your transformative journey towards a life enriched by the healing power of herbal medicine.

Just as herbal medicine has profoundly inspired and empowered my life, as we move through this book together, I express my deepest hope that the information found herein may serve as *your* inspiration and empowerment. I am deeply thankful for your trust in allowing me to accompany you. Together, let us embark on this journey to discover the nurturing power of nature and the life of health and wellness that awaits us all.

With warmth and gratitude, thank you.

Rami Archer

CHAPTER 1
THE ETERNAL WEAVE: HERBAL MEDICINE'S JOURNEY THROUGH TIME AND TRADITION

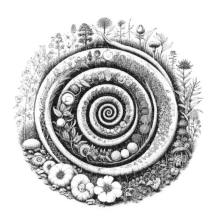

T he rich tapestry of herbal medicine weaves itself throughout the labyrinth of history. This discipline, as old as humanity itself, has been the cornerstone of healing practices across civilizations. It is a testament to the endurance and timelessness of the symbiotic relationship between humans and the natural world.

The genesis story of herbal medicine is a tale not of discovery but of intrinsic connection. Earth had provided remedies for ailments long before anyone formalized the concept of medicine.

1.1 THE ROOTS OF HERBAL MEDICINE: FROM ANCIENT CIVILIZATIONS TO TODAY

Ancient civilizations like Egypt, China, and Greece contributed significantly to the philosophical and architectural domains and were instrumental in developing herbal medicine. Their deep understanding of the natural world allowed them to harness the medicinal properties of plants, paving the way for future generations. For example, the Ebers Papyrus of Egypt extensively documents over 850 plant-based remedies, while China's seminal Huangdi Neijing integrates herbal medicine with holistic health principles, emphasizing balance and energy. Similarly, the teachings of Hippocrates in Greece highlight the importance of nature in healing, advocating for the use of dietary and herbal treatments. These civilizations advanced their medical knowledge and laid the groundwork for herbal medicine globally.

Trade routes such as the Silk Road, which connected China to the Mediterranean, greatly facilitated the exchange of herbal knowledge between these ancient cultures. This exchange enabled the blending and evolution of medicinal practices, as wisdom from the East was shared with and adapted by the West, enriching global medicinal knowledge. In the contemporary era, this ancient wisdom continues to be validated by scientific research, with numerous studies confirming the effectiveness of traditional remedies, such as ginger for nausea and turmeric for its anti-inflammatory properties. Integrating ancient herbal practices with modern medical research offers a holistic approach to healthcare, highlighting herbal medicine's timeless relevance and adaptability in promoting human health and wellness.

1.2 HERBAL INTEGRATION: BRINGING HERBAL PRACTICES INTO CONTEMPORARY MEDICINE

Reflect on the last time you sipped a cup of peppermint tea to soothe an upset stomach or applied aloe vera to a burn. These simple acts are more than home remedies—they are practices rooted in the ancient herbal medicine tradition. The invisible omnipresence of such remedies in our daily lives underscores herbal medicine's enduring importance and suggests many people already engage in the practice without realizing it. Despite advancements in medical science, the wisdom of our ancestors continues to find relevance in our modern world.

While herbal and modern medicine do not conflict, herbal medicine can offer a holistic alternative in an age when the side effects of synthetic drugs and the impersonal nature of modern healthcare can sometimes disillusion patients. It summons us with the promise of healing aligning with the body's natural rhythms, encouraging a partnership with nature to pursue health and wellness. Individuals increasingly seek ways to control their health and fitness they can trust, turning to herbal remedies to *supplement* conventional treatments with natural alternatives.

Integrating herbal practice into contemporary medicine is not a regression but an evolution—a harmonization of tradition and science. Its efficacy is evident in the growing number of hospitals and clinics incorporating herbal remedies into their treatment plans and the expanding research funding for herbal medicine; this reflects a broader shift towards holistic health, a movement driven by a desire for treatments that align with a holistic view of health—

one that considers physical, emotional, and spiritual health and well-being.

1.3 THE RENAISSANCE OF HERBAL MEDICINE IN THE 21ST CENTURY

At the dawn of the 21st century, herbal medicine has witnessed a significant revival, marked by a shift towards more natural and holistic health practices. A growing disenchantment with the impersonal nature of modern healthcare systems and an increasing awareness of the adverse effects associated with synthetic drugs primarily drive this resurgence. As people become more conscious of these issues, there's a noticeable trend toward integrating herbal remedies with conventional medical treatments. This movement is not merely a nostalgic embrace of ancient methods but a rational response to the limitations inherent in current medical paradigms, emphasizing a comprehensive approach that includes physical, emotional, and spiritual well-being.

Scientific research has played a pivotal role in reinforcing the validity of herbal medicine, providing hard evidence that supports the efficacy of various herbal remedies. Research institutions worldwide have delved into the medicinal properties of plants traditionally used in herbal treatments, bringing empirical data to what was once considered mere folklore. For example, studies validating the anti-inflammatory properties of turmeric and the stress-relief benefits of ashwagandha have played a crucial role in increasing the acceptance of these herbs within the scientific community. This acknowledgment has spurred the integration of herbal treatments into mainstream medical settings, where medical professionals increasingly view them as viable complements to pharmaceutical interventions.

Despite the positive momentum, incorporating herbal medicine into mainstream healthcare faces significant challenges, mainly regulating and standardizing herbal products. The natural variability in how plants are grown and processed complicates the consistency and safety of herbal remedies. Unlike pharmaceuticals, where active ingredients are isolated and dosages meticulously controlled, herbal treatments can vary widely in composition. This lack of standardization raises concerns about their safety, efficacy, and reliability, which remains a significant barrier to their full acceptance by the medical community. However, as consumer demand for natural health products grows, the industry is adopting stricter quality control and more rigorous product testing, promising a future where herbal medicine integrates more seamlessly into contemporary healthcare practices.

1.4 SCIENCE MEETS TRADITION: VALIDATING AND PRESERVING ANCIENT WISDOM

Integrating modern scientific methods with ancient herbal traditions represents a harmonious fusion, enhancing our understanding of natural healing. Rigorous scientific examination, through methods like phytochemical analysis and clinical trials, validates the efficacy of herbal medicine. For example, studies have shown St. John's wort effectively treats mild to moderate depression with fewer side effects than conventional antidepressants, and the discovery of artemisinin from Artemisia annua has revolutionized malaria treatment. Preserving traditional herbal knowledge through ethnobotanical studies, oral history projects, and partnerships with indigenous communities is crucial to maintaining this rich heritage. These efforts protect cultural heritage and fuel research to unlock new remedies for pressing health challenges, highlighting herbal medicine's enduring relevance and potential in modern science.

1.5 THE PHILOSOPHY OF HEALING: UNDERSTANDING THE HOLISTIC APPROACH

The holistic healing philosophy is gaining prominence, marking a shift from traditional medicine's focus on symptom management to a broader view of health. This approach treats the body as an integrated ecosystem, emphasizing the interconnectedness of physical, emotional, and spiritual health and well-being. Herbal medicine is crucial, utilizing natural substances to support the body's healing capabilities. Herbs serve as treatments and integral parts of a preventive health regimen, fostering continuous wellness. This proactive care emphasizes sustained health over-reactive disease treatment. Regularly using adaptogenic herbs like ashwagandha supports stress management, mental clarity, and emotional stability, helping maintain a balanced internal environment. Preparing and consuming herbal remedies also provides a reflective, spiritual practice, deepening one's connection to nature. As more people adopt this holistic approach, herbal medicine proves its timeless value, offering natural solutions that remain effective through the ages.

CHAPTER 2

DECIPHERING NATURE'S PHARMACY: THE WHAT, HOW, AND WHY OF HERBAL HEALING

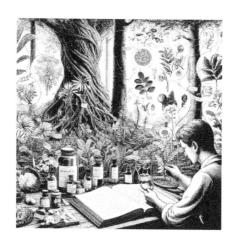

A mid the din of life's daily hustle, the subtle whisper of nature's lore often goes unnoticed. Yet, in the humblest of leaves and the most unassuming of roots lies an intricate compendium of and capacity for healing that predates the annals of recorded history. This chapter unveils the alchemy of herbal medicine—the complicated dance between plants' biochemical treasures and the complex human body systems they seek to heal. We will explore in depth the *what,* the *how*, and the awe-inspiring *why* behind nature's healing mechanisms, illuminating science that underpins herbal medicine and celebrating the profound depth of knowledge that comes from observing, studying, and honoring the natural world.

2.1 THE SCIENCE BEHIND HERBAL MEDICINE: HOW PLANTS HEAL

Herbal medicine relies on the intricate chemistry of phytochemicals, diverse bioactive compounds derived from plants that interact profoundly with human physiology. These compounds include alkaloids, flavonoids, and terpenoids, each possessing unique molecular structures that trigger specific therapeutic responses within the body. For example, the alkaloids found in dandelion roots naturally stimulate digestive secretions, a process that mirrors the body's innate response to the anticipation of food. This phytochemical activation helps the body prepare and optimize digestion, showcasing the natural integration of plant-based substances with human biological processes.

The specific interactions of these phytochemicals illustrate a form of natural alchemy. Flavonoids, for instance, are known for their potent antioxidant properties, scavenging free radicals from the body to reduce oxidative stress and bolster immune health. Terpenoids play a critical role in modulating inflammation and enhancing mood, often by interacting with neurotransmitter systems or influencing cellular signaling pathways. Phytochemicals in herbal medicine actively engage in a silent dialogue with the human body's cells, tailoring each plant compound to evoke and support natural healing processes that promote overall health and well-being.

Mechanism of Action: Nature's Pharmacodynamics

The interaction between herbal remedies and the human body is a symphony of cellular communications. Specifically, plants' phytochemicals mimic, enhance, and inhibit the actions of endogenous molecules, modulating biological pathways to promote healing. Consider the vibrant constituent of turmeric, curcumin, which intricately interacts with over 160 potential molecular targets in the body, exhibiting anti-inflammatory, antioxidant, and neuroprotective effects. This broad impact spectrum illustrates the holistic nature of herbal healing: traditional medicine addresses symptoms and, more importantly, the range of underlying imbalances that give the symptoms rise.

Phytochemicals and Their Benefits

According to " Science Direct," a website that provides access to an extensive bibliographic database of scientific and medical publications, some of the common phytochemicals are — Carotenoids, Phytosterols, Phytosterols, Polyphenols, Glucosinolates, Phytoestrogen, Terpenoids, Fibers, Polysaccharides, and Saponins. "Science Direct" lists their corresponding sources and benefits, offering readers a quick reference guide to the healing power and biochemical diversity hidden in plain sight in their gardens and kitchens.

Phytochemicals Sources Health Benefits References:

1. Phytochemical: Carotenoids

- *Sources: Carrots, tomatoes, parsley, orange and green leafy vegetables, chenopods, fenugreek, spinach, cabbage, radish, turnips*
- *Health Benefits: Antioxidants protect against uterine, prostate, colorectal, lung, and digestive tract cancers*

2. Phytochemical: Phytosterols

- *Sources: Vegetables, nuts, fruits, seeds*
- *Health Benefits: Suppress the growth of diverse tumors cell lines via initiation of apoptosis and concomitant arrest of cells in the G1 phase of the cell cycle*

3. Phytochemical: Limonoids

- *Sources: Citrus fruits*
- *Health Benefits: Inhibiting phase I enzymes and inducing phase II detoxification enzymes in liver, provide protection to lung tissue. Detoxify enzymes*

4. Phytochemical: Polyphenols

➤**Flavonoids**
➤**Isoflavonoids**
➤**Anthocyanidins**

- *Sources: Fruits, vegetables, cereals, beverages, legumes, chocolates, oilseeds*
- *Health Benefits: Action against free radicals, free radicals mediated cellular signaling, inflammation, allergies, platelet aggregation, and hepatotoxins*

5. Phytochemical: Glucosinolates

- *Sources: Cruciferous vegetables*
- *Health Benefits: Protection against cancer of colon, rectum, and stomach*

6. *Phytochemical: Phytoestrogen*

- *Sources: Legumes, berries, whole grains, cereals, red wine, peanuts, red grapes*
- *Health Benefits: Protection against bone loss and heart disease, cardiovascular diseases, breast and uterine cancers*

7. *Phytochemical: Terpenoids (Isoprenoids)*

- *Sources: Mosses, liverworts, algae, lichens, mushrooms*
- *Health Benefits: Antimicrobial, antiparasitic, antiviral, antiallergic, anti-inflammatory, chemotherapeutic, antihyperglycemic, antispasmodic*

8. *Phytochemical: Fibers*

- *Sources: Fruits and vegetables (green leafy), oats*
- *Health Benefits: Reduces blood cholesterol, cardiovascular disease*

9. *Phytochemical: Polysaccharides*

- *Sources: Fruits and vegetables*
- *Health Benefits: Antimicrobial, antiparasitic, antiviral, antiallergic, anti-inflammatory, lowering serum, enhances defense mechanisms*

10. Phytochemical: Saponins

- *Sources: Oats, leaves, flowers, and green fruits of tomato*
- *Health Benefits: Protection against pathogens, antimicrobial, anti-inflammatory, antiulcer agent*

Dissecting the science behind herbal medicine reminds us of the humility required to learn from nature. The complexity of phytochemical and human body interactions underscores the sophistication of natural remedies and thereby challenges us to look beyond the reductionist approach of isolating single active healing ingredients.

Herbal medicine invites us to embrace the holistic complexity of nature's remedies. It recognizes that the sum of any plant's parts—its unique phytochemical symphony—offers healing that transcends the capabilities of individual compounds. This chapter illuminates the science that supports herbal medicine and celebrates the profound depth of knowledge that comes from observing, studying, and honoring the natural world. As we continue to explore herbal remedies' efficacy, safety, and application considerations, let us carry forward reverence for such holistic wisdom. It has healed generations before us and holds the promise to heal countless more to come.

2.2 SAFETY FIRST: NAVIGATING HERBAL REMEDIES RESPONSIBLY

The complex chemistry and profound healing potential of plants and herbs beckon with a promise of health and rejuvenation. Yet, intertwining the ancient with the modern is understandably complex, and we cannot overstate the importance of a prudent approach to navigating this landscape. This path demands of its followers a keen awareness of inherent limitations and a steadfast commitment to responsible usage. The wisdom of the ages, coupled with contemporary understanding, serves as a guiding light—ensuring that our foray into herbal remedies enriches, rather than imperils, our quest for health and wellness.

Identifying Quality: The Pursuit of Purity and Ethics

As seekers of healing, the quest for high-quality, ethically sourced herbs is foundational to the integrity of our practice. The landscape of herbal remedies, lush with potential, is also fraught with the task of discerning the pure from the impure, the sustainably harvested from the exploitatively taken.

An herb's measures of quality—influenced by growing conditions, harvesting methods, and processing practices—directly impact its efficacy and safety. Learning to identify reputable herbal sources, an essential skill, involves:

- *Researching suppliers.*
- *Verifying their commitment to organic and sustainable practices.*
- *Ensuring their products undergo rigorous testing for purity and potency.*

Preference for suppliers who transparently share their sourcing and quality-assurance processes and practices demonstrates a commitment to personal health, the ethical dimensions of environmental stewardship, and respect for indigenous knowledge.

Safe Usage Practices: The Architecture of Dosage and Duration

Using herbal remedies safely requires building on the twin pillars of dosage and duration. Unlike conventional medications with precisely calibrated dosages, the potency of herbal remedies can vary due to species variety, plant part used, and preparation method. An informed approach begins with adhering to dosages recommended by empirical evidence and traditional use, guided by healthcare professionals who can adjust dosing based on individual responses to minimize risks. Awareness of the appropriate duration of use is equally important, as some herbs may be beneficial in the short term but harmful if taken too long. Achieving a dynamic balance between dosage and duration, tailored to the individual's unique constitution and health conditions, ensures precise and careful harnessing of the healing potential of herbs.

When to Seek Professional Help: The Path of Collaboration

Embarking on the path of herbal medicine is a collaborative journey that you should undertake with the guidance of healthcare professionals well-versed in conventional and herbal therapeutics. Consulting with trusted practitioners is particularly crucial for individuals with chronic conditions, those on prescription medications, and pregnant or breastfeeding women. These professionals can offer valuable insights into potential herb-drug interactions, assess the suitability of specific herbs based on your unique health history, and monitor your progress to make necessary adjustments. This partnership, grounded in trust and mutual respect, ensures your exploration of herbal remedies is safe and effective. A responsible approach to herbal medicine involves recognizing limitations, committing to quality, adhering to safe usage practices, and seeking professional advice. By following a path of prudence and collaboration, you can achieve excellent health and well-being while harmonizing with the natural world's healing potential.

2.3 HERBAL QUALITY AND SOURCING: FINDING THE BEST INGREDIENTS

Determining herbal quality and navigating the herbal sourcing web requires a discerning eye, attuned not merely to the vibrant allure of nature's bounty but also to subtleties that distinguish the exceptional from the mediocre. This pursuit needs to be more transactional. It's a conscientious endeavor in which choices ripple through ecosystems, communities, and the fabric of traditional knowledge. Guidelines emerge as beacons, guiding enthusiasts and healers alike in their quest for ingredients that embody purity, efficacy, and respect for the natural and cultural landscapes from which they originate.

Prioritizing Quality: How Herbs are Grown and Harvested

The quest for high-quality, sustainable herbs mandates vigilance and beckons a preference for organically grown herbs. Such plants are free from the taint of chemical pesticides and fertilizers, ensuring the healing essence of each leaf and root remains unblemished. This reverence also extends to harvesting methods, favoring practices that sustain, rather than deplete, plant populations and habitat health. Certifications such as Fair Trade and Rainforest Alliance have emerged as assurance symbols, indicating that designated herbs uphold ecological and social integrity standards in their sourcing.

Sourcing and purchasing considerations: A responsibility to the environment

Ethical considerations in sourcing herbs are pivotal in herbal medicine, emphasizing a profound respect for nature and the diverse cultures that have nurtured these remedies through the ages. The act of foraging, a method as ancient as humanity itself, carries a critical responsibility to engage with the environment conscientiously. Herbalists who adhere to the "Leave No Trace" philosophy are encouraged to harvest only the herbs needed and to do so in a manner that minimizes impact, ensuring the continued vitality of plant populations. This practice extends to respecting the land, requiring permissions where necessary, and avoiding areas of cultural significance to indigenous groups. Such ethical foraging ensures that herbal practices contribute positively to the conservation of plant species, particularly those rare or endangered, fostering a sustainable relationship with our planet's botanical resources.

Additionally, you must rigorously verify the integrity of commercially purchased herbal products to maintain the efficacy and safety of herbal medicine. Consumers and practitioners must scrutinize product labels for organic certification and the absence of unnecessary additives, ensuring that the herbs contain active constituents at therapeutic concentrations. This level of diligence is crucial in an era where transparency is accessible, allowing us to investigate the origins of our herbal products and the practices of the suppliers. By choosing suppliers who adhere to ethical cultivation and harvesting standards, individuals support sustainable practices and honor the traditional wisdom embedded in herbal medicine. This thoughtful approach to sourcing and consumption safeguards the potency of herbal remedies. It upholds a narrative of respect and responsibility that bridges our past with a more sustainable future, wherein healing and environmental stewardship are inextricably linked.

CHAPTER 3

CONFRONTING THE HEAVY HITTERS: HERBAL REMEDIES FOR CHRONIC CONDITIONS

Integrating herbal remedies into contemporary healthcare systems marks a significant advancement in managing chronic health conditions. As modern research continues to validate the benefits of herbs like turmeric for its anti-inflammatory properties, ginger for digestive health, and boswellia for joint pain relief, the potential of these natural solutions to enhance traditional medical treatments is becoming increasingly apparent. This shift is not just a resurgence of ancient practices but is grounded in rigorous scientific evaluation, confirming the role of herbal remedies as effective complementary therapies. Incorporating herbs such as cinnamon for blood sugar control, eleuthero for increased vitality, and cordyceps for improved respiratory and kidney function offers a personalized, less invasive approach to healthcare. This trend aligns with the current healthcare landscape, with a growing preference for treatments that address the symptoms, promote overall health and well-being, and minimize side effects. As research advances, herbal medicine will play a crucial role in holistic health strategies, offering a sustainable and effective option for managing chronic diseases and supporting patients' long-term wellness.

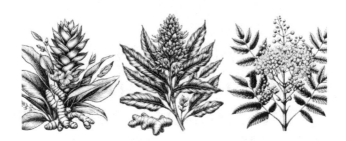

3.1 EQUALIZING INFLAMMATION WITH TURMERIC, GINGER, AND BOSWELLIA

In the intricate web of human health and wellness, inflammation is a paradoxical force—it can be both a guardian and a harbinger of poor health, depending on context and individual circumstances. This paradoxical force intrinsically weaves into our health and well-being. This duality calls for a nuanced healing approach that honors the body's innate wisdom while gently guiding it back to equilibrium. Enter the realm of anti-inflammatory herbs, where turmeric, ginger, and boswellia reign as venerable healers, their roots and rhizomes steeped in the wisdom of centuries of medicinal use. These botanicals, armed with compounds capable of quelling the fires of inflammation, offer a holistic avenue for managing chronic conditions that elude the grasp of conventional medicine.

Understanding Inflammation

At its core, inflammation is the body's alarm system, its guard—a call-to-arms response against invaders and injury. Yet, when this system malfunctions, when the alarm bell refuses to silence, the guard turns into the aggressor. Ensuing chronic inflammation lays the groundwork for severe, chronic ailments, from arthritis to heart disease. The complexity of the inflammation state and the cascade of biochemical events it triggers underscores the need for interventions that modulate the body's inflammatory response and restore the delicate balance of this protective mechanism.

Herbs and Their Anti-inflammatory Actions

Turmeric, Ginger, and Boswellia stand as herbal soldiers at the forefront of the fight against chronic inflammation, each wielding a unique arsenal of phytochemicals. If inflammation is an overflowing pipe, turmeric turns off the water valve; its curcuminoids, renowned for their potent anti-inflammatory and antioxidant properties, inhibit key enzymes in the inflammation pathway, akin to turning off a water valve to prevent overflow. If inflammation is a tumultuous region on the brink of war, ginger, with its gingerols and shogaols, suppresses pro-inflammatory compounds, much like a skilled diplomat negotiating peace in that tumultuous landscape. And if inflammation is the invading army, boswellia, through its boswellic acids, blocks the production of leukotrienes. These substances exacerbate inflammatory activity, acting as a shield against the onslaught.

Practical Applications

The integration of these anti-inflammatory herbs into daily meals transforms the act of eating into a therapeutic ritual. Consider infusing turmeric into a morning smoothie, with a pinch of black pepper (which enhances curcumin absorption) becoming a vibrant elixir to start the day. Grating fresh ginger into a warm bowl of soup or steeped into tea is a comforting inflammation remedy, its spicy notes dancing on the palate. Though less common in culinary traditions, you can incorporate boswellia into your diet through quality supplements that preserve its healing essence.

Considerations and Interactions

While the benefits of these herbs are manifold, it is nevertheless paramount to be mindful of approaching their use. Risks of interactions with pharmaceutical medications, particularly blood thinners and anticoagulants, require patients to engage in a preliminary dialogue with healthcare professionals. This dialogue ensures that integrating these anti-inflammatory herbal remedies into one's regimen harmonizes with existing treatments. The nuances of each individual's health landscape, with its unique contours and challenges, magnify inflammation's role in health and well-being and demand a personalized approach that tailors these herbs to achieve optimal health outcomes.

In the realm of chronic conditions, where the quest for relief often leads through a frustrating labyrinth of treatments and interventions, anti-inflammatory herbs emerge as beacons of hope. In their gentle yet formidable capacity to modulate inflammation, turmeric, ginger, and boswellia offer a path to wellness paved with the wisdom of nature. This path, illuminated by centuries of medicinal use and validated by contemporary research, holds the promise of healing and harmony, rekindling the ancient dialogue between humankind and the botanical world.

For further reading, you can explore more details through the following links:

Turmeric and Its Antioxidant Curcumin:

https://www.verywellhealth.com/turmeric-curcumin-benefits-7110668

Health of Ginger root

https://www.verywellhealth.com/ginger-health-uses-nutrition-and-more-7487136

Boswellia: A Supplement to Relieve Inflammation:

https://www.verywellhealth.com/the-health-benefits-of-boswellia-89549

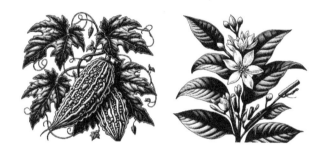

3.2 MANAGING DIABETES WITH BITTER MELON AND CINNAMON

Bitter Melon and Cinnamon are increasingly recognized for their efficacy in managing diabetes, a condition marked by the body's inability to regulate blood sugar effectively. These natural remedies, rooted in traditional medicine, significantly impact glucose regulation. Bitter Melon is known for compounds like charantin, vicine, and polypeptide-p, which mimic insulin by promoting glucose uptake and metabolism, thus enhancing glycemic control. Similarly, cinnamon contains cinnamaldehyde and polyphenolic polymers that improve insulin sensitivity and reduce fasting blood sugar levels, aligning closely with the mechanisms of modern diabetes medications. Integrating these herbs into diabetes management strategies exemplifies a growing trend toward embracing holistic and natural therapeutic options alongside conventional treatments, offering a comprehensive approach that targets the symptoms, minimizes side effects, and promotes overall metabolic health. This fusion of ancient herbal wisdom with contemporary scientific validation underscores the potential of natural therapies to contribute effectively to the broader healthcare spectrum, particularly in chronic disease management like diabetes.

Practical Applications

Incorporating bitter melon and cinnamon into the diet as part of a diabetes management plan is a nuanced approach that requires careful consideration of how these ingredients are prepared and consumed. Bitter Melon, known for its ability to assist in blood sugar regulation due to its bioactive compounds, can be integrated directly into meals. People commonly use it as a vegetable in various dishes—its unique bitter flavor makes it a popular addition to stir-fries, soups, and salads in many Asian cuisines. For those who find the taste challenging, bitter melon is also available in extract and supplement form, which provides a concentrated dose of its beneficial properties without the intense flavor. When starting with bitter melon, it's advisable to begin with smaller doses to assess tolerance and gradually increase to the optimal dosage as recommended.

Conversely, cinnamon offers a more universally appealing flavor, making it an easy and delightful addition to a wide range of dishes. Its sweet and warming taste enhances the flavor profile of breakfast cereals, baked goods, and even savory dishes. Moreover, cinnamon can be brewed into a comforting tea or blended into smoothies, providing a versatile and enjoyable method to incorporate its glucose-modulating benefits regularly. Consistent consumption is the key to effectively using both bitter melon and cinnamon, as maintaining regular levels of these substances in the body is crucial to exert their therapeutic effects. Thus, integrating these natural ingredients into daily meals not only contributes to managing diabetes but also adds nutritional and flavor diversity to the diet.

Considerations and Interactions

Effective diabetes management requires a balanced approach, where integrating natural remedies like bitter melon and cinnamon works in conjunction with, rather than as a substitute for, conventional treatments. These herbs, known for their glucose-regulating properties, should be considered complementary additions to existing medical regimens rather than standalone solutions. Open communication with healthcare providers is essential to ensure these natural supplements are beneficial and do not interfere with prescribed medications. This dialogue ensures that incorporating bitter melon and cinnamon aligns with one's overall treatment plan and considers any potential interactions with other drugs.

Regular monitoring of blood sugar levels is another critical aspect of managing diabetes, especially when introducing new elements like herbal remedies. By diligently tracking glucose fluctuations, individuals and their healthcare providers can observe the effects of bitter melon and cinnamon on their metabolic health. This ongoing data collection provides a reliable basis for making informed dosage adjustments or dietary strategies tailored to the individual's needs and responses. Such a collaborative and informed approach not only enhances the efficacy of diabetes management but also respects the complex nature of the disease and the unique physiological makeup of each person. This personalized pathway, supported by modern medicine and traditional herbal practices, offers a comprehensive strategy for achieving and maintaining optimal metabolic health.

For further reading, you can explore more details through the following links:

Bitter Melon: Benefits and Nutrition

https://www.verywellhealth.com/bitter-melon-benefits-and-nutrition-7505756

Evidenced-Based Health Benefits of Cinnamon

https://www.verywellhealth.com/cinnamon-7505730

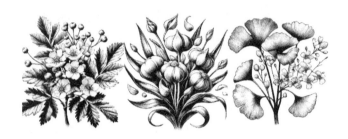

3.3 HERBAL APPROACHES TO CARDIOVASCULAR HEALTH

In the intricate web of cardiovascular health, where every heartbeat narrates the tale of life's fragility and resilience, hawthorn, garlic, and ginkgo biloba emerge from nature's pharmacopeia as stalwarts of vitality. People have revered these herbs through the ages for their life-sustaining properties. They offer a beacon of hope, illuminating a path to heart wellness that transcends conventional paradigms. Their capacity to fortify heart health, enhance circulation, and shield against the ravages of oxidative stress reflects a deep alignment with the body's natural rhythms, a testament to their enduring legacy as guardians of the human heart.

Herbs and Their Cardiovascular Actions

The mechanism through which these herbal allies bestow their benefits upon the cardiovascular system is via a symphony of biochemical interactions, a harmonious convergence of nature's ingenuity, and the body's inherent wisdom. If a diseased heart is an out-of-tune piano, hawthorn acts directly on the heart's muscular fibers to enhance the force and efficiency of heartbeats. With its rich tapestry of flavonoids and oligomeric proanthocyanidins, hawthorn strengthens the force and efficiency of heartbeats, thus optimizing the heart's ability to pump blood. This action, akin to tuning a grand piano to produce the most resonant melodies, ensures that every note the heart plays contributes to the symphony of overall health and well-being. Garlic is its skilled sculptor, leveraging its potent allicin content to operate on the arterial system. It gently dilates blood vessels and reduces the pressure exerted upon the heart's walls, a crucial factor in preventing hypertension. And if the body is a thirsty plant, ginkgo biloba acts as its watering can; famous for its ginkgolides, ginkgo enhances microcirculation to ensure that blood's life-sustaining cargo nourishes even the most remote regions of the body. In their unique ways, this trio mitigates oxidative stress, a silent thief of vitality, thus shielding the heart and vessels from the insidious advancing of age and disease.

Practical applications

Crafting a heart-healthy herbal regimen from these botanicals requires an approach that is both art and science, a delicate balancing act that honors the individuality of each body. Initiating this regimen with hawthorn, one might incorporate it into daily rituals via teas or tinctures, starting with modest doses that can be gradually adjusted, allowing the body to acclimate to hawthorn's strengthening embrace. Garlic, in its culinary versatility, enriches a plethora of dishes, from the simplicity of roasted vegetables to the complexity of hearty stews, infusing meals with its protective essence; for those seeking garlic's protective benefits without its intense aroma, aged supplements offer a palatable alternative. You can most readily find ginkgo biloba in capsule or liquid extract form; when including it to complement this regimen, you must carefully consider individual needs and existing health conditions. This holistic approach, woven into the fabric of daily life, transforms routine into ritual, each meal, each sip, a reaffirmation of life's potential for renewal and healing.

Considerations and Interactions

Navigating heart health as one adopts this herbal regimen becomes not just a practice but a profound act of self-awareness. Regular consultations with healthcare providers ensure that the integration of these herbs synergizes with one's unique physiological narrative, adapting and evolving in response to the body's cues. This dynamic process adapts with ongoing health assessments, mirroring the natural world's adaptability and testifying to the fluidity and resilience that characterize life. In this dynamic context, blood pressure readings, cholesterol levels, and heart rate variability data serve as markers on the map of heart health, guiding the optimization of the herbal regimen to support the heart's journey toward optimal function.

For further reading, you can explore more details through the following links:

Hawthorn: Benefits and Nutrition
https://www.verywellhealth.com/the-benefits-of-hawthorn-89057

What Is Allicin? Garlic's Heart-Health Booster
https://www.verywellhealth.com/the-benefits-of-allicin-88606

The Health Benefits and Side Effects of Ginkgo Biloba
https://www.verywellmind.com/ginkgo-what-should-you-know-about-it-88329

3.4 ADAPTOGENS FOR LONG-TERM STRESS AND FATIGUE

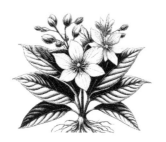 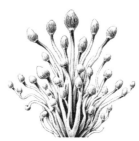

In the relentless ebb and flow of modern existence, where stress and fatigue all too often lay siege to our health and well-being, adaptogens stand as ancient sentinels, offering sanctuary from the storm. These botanical guardians possess an extraordinary capacity to modulate the body's stress response, providing hope for us navigating the tumultuous waters of chronic stress and fatigue. Among the pantheon of adaptogens, eleuthero, and cordyceps emerge as potent allies, their roots, and spores deeply entwined with the fabric of traditional healing practices across diverse cultures. Their unique profiles offer a nuanced approach to stress management, addressing the multifaceted nature of chronic stress and fatigue with grace and efficacy.

Herbs and Their Stress-Relieving Actions

Eleuthero sometimes referred to as "Siberian Ginseng", and Cordyceps are esteemed in herbal medicine for their unique abilities to enhance physical and mental resilience without the drawbacks of stimulants like caffeine. Eleuthero supports the body's stress response by optimizing adrenal gland function, which regulates hormone production and maintains energy levels through balanced stress hormone secretion. This function helps preserve the body's energy for sustained endurance and mental clarity. Similarly, people celebrate cordyceps for its ability to increase ATP (*adenosine triphosphate*) production and improve oxygen utilization, which boosts physical stamina and cognitive functions. The increase in ATP production makes it particularly beneficial for individuals experiencing fatigue that affects both the body and mind. Together, these adaptogens offer a natural, efficient way to enhance metabolic efficiency and overall vitality, proving invaluable in managing stress and fatigue holistically.

Practical Applications

Incorporating these adaptogens into the rhythms of daily life necessitates a tailored approach, one that respects personal preferences and lifestyle nuances. For eleuthero, integration takes many forms. You might begin with morning infusions of the herb's earthy tones blending seamlessly with the tea ritual, setting a foundation of calm and resilience for the day ahead. Alternatively, tinctures or capsules provide a convenient means of consumption, particularly for those whose mornings are a whirlwind of activity. With its versatile application, cordyceps can be woven into the diet in powder form, enriching smoothies, soups, or even coffee. It offers a subtle lift that carries one through the day without the precipitous crash associated with traditional stimulants.

Considerations and Interactions

Yet, the true art of employing adaptogens for stress and fatigue lies not in their isolated use but in their integration into a holistic stress management strategy. This strategy acknowledges that proper recovery from chronic stress involves a mosaic of rest, nutrition, movement, and mindfulness practices, with adaptogens serving as one piece of this larger puzzle. Eleuthero and Cordyceps, while their role alleviates symptoms of stress and fatigue, also underscores the importance of cultivating practices that replenish the body *and* spirit. In short, such an herbal regimen will only be effective when you prioritize quality sleep, engage in activities that ground and center the mind, and nurture the body with nourishing and revitalizing foods.

In this balanced approach, adaptogens act not as crutches but as catalysts, encouraging the body to access its innate capacity for resilience and vitality. This balanced approach reminds us that, in the quest for health and well-being, the wisdom of nature serves not as a substitute but as a complement to the inherent knowledge of self-care. By fostering a symbiotic relationship with these herbal allies, we learn to navigate the currents of stress and fatigue with grace, emerging not only stronger but more attuned to the rhythms of our nature.

For further reading, you can explore more details through the following links:

Potential Health Benefits of Eleuthero
https://www.verywellhealth.com/health-benefits-of-eleuthero-89449

What Are the Health Benefits of Cordyceps Supplements?
https://www.verywellhealth.com/benefits-of-cordyceps-89441

CHAPTER 4
THE ALCHEMY OF RELIEF: NATURAL REMEDIES FOR PAIN MANAGEMENT

The pursuit of effective pain management has led many to embrace natural remedies, which offer relief while aligning with the body's natural processes. Historically and scientifically supported botanicals like willow bark, jamaican dogwood, california poppy, kratom, and kava serve as key players in this arena. Willow Bark, known as "nature's aspirin," provides pain relief through salicin, akin to salicylic acid. At the same time, traditional Caribbean medicine utilizes jamaican dogwood for its strong analgesic properties against nerve pain and migraines. California Poppy contributes mild sedative and analgesic effects, offering a non-addictive solution to improve sleep and alleviate discomfort. On the other hand, kratom and kava, despite their controversy, are respected in their native regions for treating pain and anxiety, illustrating the delicate balance of benefit and safety in pain management. These plants mitigate physical pain and incorporate emotional and psychological healing, demonstrating a holistic approach that modern medicine is beginning to acknowledge and integrate, enhancing overall health and well-being.

4.1 WILLOW BARK: NATURE'S ASPIRIN FOR PAIN AND INFLAMMATION

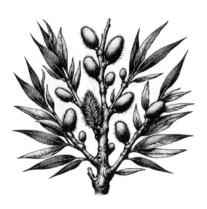

Willow bark has long stood as a pillar of natural remedy, its profound efficacy woven deeply into the tapestry of medical history and human endurance. The celebration of willow bark has been going on for thousands of years; from the ancient Sumerians to the Greeks under Hippocrates, they utilized willow bark to soothe fevers and alleviate aches. It carries its legacy into contemporary times as a natural alternative to synthetic analgesics, earning it the nickname "nature's aspirin." This remarkable herb not only underscores the continuity of herbal medicine across centuries but also highlights the evolving understanding and appreciation of its mechanisms—salicin's conversion into salicylic acid within the body mirrors the effects of modern drugs but through natural processes. As we seek holistic approaches to health, willow bark remains a cornerstone for innovation in pain relief and inflammation management, embodying a blend of tradition and modern science that advocates for a balanced approach to physical health and well-being. This synergy invites a deeper exploration of other traditional remedies, encouraging a broader acceptance and integration of natural healing practices in modern medicine.

Practical applications

Willow Bark truly transcends time as a natural remedy for pain and inflammation. It represents the profound connection between the physical body and the natural world, reaffirming the value of traditional knowledge for shaping contemporary approaches to health and wellness. Willow bark is a versatile natural remedy available in various forms, including powder, liquid, capsules, and teas. Using willow bark effectively for pain relief hinges on understanding its dosage and preparation methods. For those preferring to use willow bark in tea form, it is essential to source high-quality, dried willow bark from reliable health stores or online herbal suppliers. It is common to use approximately 2-3 grams of willow bark per cup to prepare the tea. Begin by boiling water, then add the willow bark and allow it to simmer for about 15 minutes. This simmering process is crucial as it helps to effectively release the active compound, salicin, from the bark. This preparation method ensures the therapeutic properties of willow bark are preserved and effective when ingested. The advisable initial dose of willow bark tea is generally one cup daily, especially for new users, to monitor the body's response to salicin. If well-tolerated, you can adjust the dosage based on individual needs and recommendations from a healthcare provider.

Considerations and Interactions

For individuals considering willow bark for pain management, especially those with aspirin allergies or who are on blood-thinning medications, understanding the similarities between salicin and aspirin is crucial. These similarities suggest that salicin might provoke similar adverse reactions as aspirin, thus necessitating caution. Consulting with healthcare professionals is essential before incorporating willow bark into their regimen. This step ensures that patients can balance the potential benefits of willow bark against the possible risks. Such consultations safeguard health by preventing adverse interactions and empower individuals by equipping them with the knowledge needed to make informed decisions. Tailoring willow bark to fit one's unique health profile enhances its efficacy and safety, reinforcing the value of personalized medicine in natural health practices. This approach highlights the importance of integrating traditional remedies with modern medical advice to achieve the best health outcomes.

For further reading, you can explore more details through the following link:

Willow Bark

https://www.drugs.com/npc/willow-bark.html

4.2 JAMAICAN DOGWOOD: A POTENT REMEDY FOR NERVE PAIN

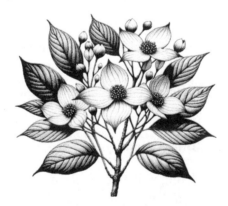

Jamaican Dogwood is a notable standout in the vast landscape of herbal remedies that address pain management, particularly its effectiveness against nerve pain. Indigenous to the lush environments of the Caribbean and specific areas of Florida, people have utilized this natural remedy for centuries, valuing it for its potent analgesic properties. Its application in traditional medicine primarily centers on alleviating intense nerve-related discomfort, such as that experienced with conditions like sciatica or fibromyalgia. The active compounds in jamaican dogwood target and modulate pain pathways, offering significant relief without the side effects commonly associated with synthetic medications and making jamaican dogwood not only a powerful tool in the natural treatment of nerve pain but also a critical component of holistic health practices, bridging the gap between traditional knowledge and modern therapeutic approaches.

Pain-relieving actions

Among the cadre of bioactive compounds, these botanical secrets, isoflavones, and rotenoids especially stand out for their analgesic prowess. These compounds interact with the central nervous system to attenuate the sharp, often debilitating sensations associated with sciatica, migraines, etc. Though incomplete, preliminary scientific research suggests that this relief may result from these compounds inhibiting pain signals at their source. This explanation offers the hope of solace to those who have found little relief for chronic pain in conventional treatments. However, according to an article from Mount Sinai, "Jamaica dogwood is not recommended for human use and should never be taken without a doctor's close supervision. Animal studies have shown that jamaica dogwood may promote sleep, relieve pain, reduce smooth muscle spasms, relieve cough, and reduce fever and inflammation. However, it is also potentially toxic."

Jamaican Dogwood

https:www.mountsinai.org/health-library/herb/jamaica-dogwood

Practical applications

A direct route of jamaican dogwood ingestion can be found in tinctures, revered for their concentrated potency, promising swift alleviation of discomfort; you can also find jamaican dogwood in liquid extract or make it into tea. Teas, conversely, provide a gentler introduction to the herb's benefits, marrying the therapeutic process with the calming ritual of tea consumption. Know that the choice between these application methods is not trivial; it reflects and necessitates a deeper understanding of your relationship with pain and your desired journey toward relief. Within this choice, efficacy finds its partner in personal comfort, ensuring that the path to pain management is as soothing as the destination. It is important to note that you should only take jamaican dogwood after consulting a healthcare professional.

Considerations and Interactions

Jamaican Dogwood, known for its potent pain-relieving properties, requires careful handling due to its potential toxicity, which can lead to symptoms like numbness and tremors, making it crucial for healthcare professionals to oversee its use. Particularly vulnerable groups such as pregnant and breastfeeding women, older adults, and those on CNS (*central nervous system*) depressants should avoid this herb due to the risk of severe side effects and adverse interactions. Moreover, you must consider ethical and environmental considerations, as jamaican dogwood, native to limited regions, is susceptible to overharvesting, threatening its survival and the ecological balance of its habitats. Adopting sustainable sourcing practices is essential to preserve this valuable botanical without compromising its cultural heritage and environmental integrity, ensuring its benefits are delivered safely and responsibly.

For further reading, you can explore more details through the following link:

Jamaican Dogwood
https://www.webmd.com/vitamins/ai/ingredientmono-529/
jamaican-dogwood

4.3 CALIFORNIA POPPY: MILD PAIN RELIEF FOR A RESTFUL SLEEP

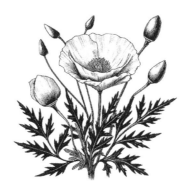

In the tranquil embrace of twilight, when the world softens and the boundaries between wakefulness and sleep blur, the california poppy emerges as a guardian of restfulness and peace.

The california poppy, a vibrant and natural herb, offers a gentle yet effective approach to pain relief, particularly when it comes to enhancing restful sleep. Known scientifically as *Eschscholzia californica*, this plant is a revered herbal remedy. Its mild sedative properties make it ideal for those seeking to alleviate discomfort and improve sleep quality without strong pharmaceuticals. As a non-addictive alternative to traditional pain medications, california poppy provides a holistic way to manage pain while fostering a peaceful night's sleep.

Pain-Relieving Actions

California poppy carries properties that gently ease pain and usher in the sanctity of sleep. This plant harbors a complex array of alkaloids within its delicate form, most notably protopine and allocryptopine. These subtle yet effective compounds navigate the delicate pathways of pain and restlessness, offering a safe, mild amelioration of discomfort and insomnia. People revere the california poppy for its gentleness. Its dual benefits include its ability to alleviate pain without the forcefulness of conventional analgesics and to smooth the passage to sleep. Unlike the potent opiates that bind heavy-handedly to the body's receptors, the poppy's alkaloids whisper to the nervous system, modulating pain perception and inducing a state of natural calm without clouding consciousness.

Practical Applications

The alchemy of transforming the california poppy into a conduit of relief and rest begins with the simplicity of preparation. A tea, steeped with reverence for the plant's potency, becomes a vessel carrying the promise of tranquility. To prepare the poppy via the tea ritual, simmer a modest measure of the dried plant in water, allowing the essence to infuse the liquid with its golden hue and therapeutic virtues. When undertaken in the quiet hour before sleep, this infusion process becomes a true meditative ritual, a moment of pause that honors the body's need for rest. On the other hand, for those seeking the convenience of encapsulated remedies or tinctures, the market also offers california poppy in these forms, ensuring its benefits are accessible to all who seek its gentle embrace.

The california poppy, while effective on its own, achieves optimal results for pain relief and sleep enhancement when incorporated into a holistic regimen that nurtures the body, mind, and spirit. This regimen includes pairing its use with mindfulness practices, choosing anti-inflammatory foods that complement the plant's benefits, and engaging in gentle physical activities like yoga or stretching before bed. Revered for its subtle yet powerful healing properties, the california poppy honors the body's natural rhythms and exemplifies the profound impact of gentle, integrative interventions for health and well-being.

Considerations and Interactions

California poppy, known for its calming and sleep-promoting properties, is a versatile tea, tincture, and capsule herb. However, you should determine the proper dosage with the guidance of a healthcare provider. While generally safe for adults, it can trigger allergic reactions such as rashes and respiratory issues in sensitive individuals. Due to limited research, pregnant or breastfeeding women should not use it without professional advice. Given the sedative qualities of california poppy, you should discontinue it at least two weeks before any surgery to avoid interactions with anesthesia and other medications.

Moreover, its effects may intensify when combined with sedatives like benzodiazepines or CNS depressants and other substances that cause drowsiness, such as valerian, kava, and melatonin. It may also lower blood pressure, posing risks when used with hypertension medications, and could interact with pain medications, including opioids, affecting their efficacy or side effects. Responsible use of california poppy requires awareness of these potential interactions and consulting a healthcare provider before beginning treatment, particularly for those with existing health conditions or on other medications.

For further reading, you can explore more details through the following link:

Poppy
https://www.drugs.com/npp/poppy.html#24362742

4.4 KRATOM AND KAVA: CONTROVERSIAL YET EFFECTIVE PAIN SOLUTIONS

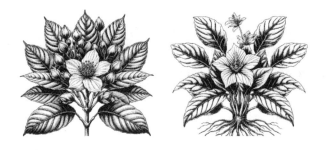

Within the diverse array of herbal remedies for pain management, kratom, and kava stand out as particularly notable yet contentious options. Both botanicals carry a rich tradition of use in their native regions, and people celebrate them for their potential therapeutic benefits. However, they also attract significant debate and scrutiny. Kratom, derived from a tree native to Southeast Asia, and kava, hailing from the Pacific Islands, sparks essential conversations about the intersection of efficacy and safety and the challenges of balancing traditional uses with modern regulatory frameworks. This complex dialogue underscores the critical need to carefully evaluate these herbal solutions' benefits and risks.

Pain-Relieving Actions

Kratom leaves harbor compounds with effects that mimic those of opiates *without* deriving from the poppy. Mitragynine and 7-hydroxymitragynine, the primary alkaloids in kratom, engage with the body's opioid receptors, alleviating severe pain with a proficiency that draws parallels to opiate medications. Yet, unlike their pharmaceutical counterparts, the effects of kratom extend beyond simple analgesia—they also touch on energy enhancement and mood elevation, aspects that have endeared them to a diverse cohort of relief seekers.

Kava, a root revered in the Pacific Islands for its ceremonial and therapeutic uses, presents a fascinating study on the dual nature of botanical remedies. Its active compounds, known as kavalactones, exhibit pronounced analgesic *and* anxiolytic properties, a dream combination for those besieged by pain intertwined with the tendrils of anxiety. The mechanism through which kava operates suggests an interaction with the central nervous system that tempers the body's stress response using gentle coaxing rather than forceful suppression. This subtle modulation allows for relief from pain and anxiety without the clouding of consciousness or diminishment of vitality, characteristics often associated with conventional comparable pharmacological interventions.

Considerations and Interactions

The use of kratom and kava in pain management is enveloped in a complex landscape of legal and safety considerations, reflecting a diverse spectrum of acceptance and restriction. Kava, with its long history, has faced regulatory scrutiny in certain countries due to potential liver toxicity risks, necessitating cautious consumption. Kratom, meanwhile, remains in a legal grey area, with ongoing debates concerning its safety and potential for dependency influencing its regulatory status, which fluctuates between being permitted and prohibited. These issues underscore the necessity for informed and responsible usage of these herbs. Individuals considering these substances for pain management must carefully weigh the benefits against the risks, starting with low doses and closely monitoring for adverse effects. Regular consultations with healthcare professionals familiar with these botanicals are crucial to ensure their use is beneficial and aligns with overall health and wellness goals. This cautious approach reflects a broader narrative of balancing efficacy and safety, tradition and regulation in the quest for effective pain and anxiety relief.

For further reading, you can explore more details through the following links:

Kratom: Weighing the Benefits and Risks
https://www.verywellhealth.com/kratom-7499659

Kava: Everything You Need to Know
https://www.verywellhealth.com/kava-uses-risks-and-more-7481255

CHAPTER 5
THE ESSENCE OF PURIFICATION: HERBS FOR DETOXIFICATION

Detoxification through herbal remedies is a practice steeped in ancient and contemporary health traditions, highlighting the essential need for the body to eliminate toxins to maintain optimal health. Herbs such as milk thistle, dandelion, burdock root, cilantro, and turmeric are among the most effective in facilitating this process, each providing unique benefits that support the body's natural cleansing and rejuvenation. Milk thistle, particularly revered for its liver-protecting properties, uses its active ingredient, silymarin, to protect liver cells from damage and promote the repair of damaged cells. Similarly, dandelion enhances liver function and aids in toxin elimination through its diuretic effects, supporting kidney health.

Expanding the scope of detoxification, burdock root works to purify the blood by removing toxins and bolstering the body with its antioxidant and anti-inflammatory properties. Cilantro offers a distinct detox path by binding to heavy metals like lead and mercury, facilitating their removal and preventing potential long-term health problems associated with heavy metal toxicity. Turmeric complements this herbal detox ensemble with its potent anti-inflammatory and antioxidant capabilities, which are crucial for liver health and fighting oxidative stress. Curcumin in turmeric boosts the production of detoxifying enzymes, enhancing overall immune function. Collectively, these herbs create a comprehensive detoxification regimen, tapping into the age-old wisdom of herbal cleansing to promote a healthier, toxin-free body naturally and holistically.

5.1 MILK THISTLE: A LIVER PROTECTOR AND DETOXIFIER

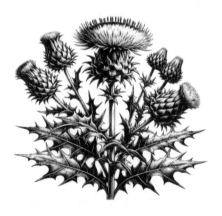

In an environment where pollutants permeate the air, water, and food, the liver functions as a crucial but often underappreciated defense mechanism. It continuously works to filter and neutralize an array of harmful substances that enter the body daily. This vital organ not only detoxifies chemicals but also metabolizes drugs, all while facilitating the body's internal cleansing processes. As such, potential toxins constantly expose the liver, potentially impairing its function over time and highlighting the need for adequate support mechanisms to maintain its health.

Enter milk thistle, a plant with remarkable protective and restorative properties for the liver, primarily due to its silymarin content. This powerful herb supports the liver's detoxification pathways, boosting its ability to flush toxins. By doing so, milk thistle not only safeguards the liver from incoming threats but also aids in the body's overall detoxification system, essential for maintaining optimal health in a polluted world. Thus, milk thistle is a potent ally in the quest for liver health, providing critical support to an organ that plays a central role in systemic detoxification and overall health and well-being.

Detoxifying Actions

Silymarin, the active compound found within milk thistle seeds, operates not merely as a shield for liver cells but also as a regenerator. Silymarin, a group of flavonoids known for their antioxidant and anti-inflammatory properties, protects liver cells by preventing the entrance of toxin-laden molecules. By stabilizing cell membranes and fostering the repair of damaged liver tissue, silymarin ensures the liver's tireless and critical resilience against the modern environment's relentless toxins. Such stabilization and regeneration can be most revolutionary for those battling liver conditions or seeking to bolster liver health.

Moreover, it promotes the regeneration of damaged liver tissue, helping to restore liver function more rapidly. Silymarin also stimulates the synthesis of proteins, which can enhance the liver's ability to repair itself following injury caused by exposure to pollutants, alcohol, and other liver-damaging substances.

Integration with Other Detox Herbs

While potent on its own, milk thistle finds synergy in the company of other detoxifying herbs that amplify its collective power to cleanse and protect. Dandelion root (see below), with its diuretic properties, complements milk thistle's liver support to facilitate the removal of toxins through the kidneys. Together, this is an example of herbs forging a coalition, marshaling the body's natural detoxification processes to fortify against the relentless siege of environmental toxins.

Milk Thistle's capacity for resilience and renewal mirrors the liver's remarkable capacity for regeneration. With its deep roots in herbal medicine, this herb offers more than support for one critical organ; it embodies the larger narrative of the body's innate ability to cleanse and heal and the power of nature to nurture and protect, a reminder of the body's enduring strength and the profound healing found in the embrace of the natural world.

Practical Applications

Milk Thistle avails itself of many forms—from capsules and tablets to liquid extracts and teas—each offering a pathway to its liver-protective benefits. The key to harnessing its potential lies in navigating these options to the modality that best resonates with your lifestyle and preferences; for those inclined towards the tea ritual, steeping milk thistle seeds or leaves becomes a daily act of self-care. Meanwhile, capsules provide the advantage of measurability, which is particularly attractive for those seeking to track specific dosages. (The consensus here on optimal dosage suggests an adjustable range based on individual needs and the severity of liver concerns, underscoring the importance of personalization.)

Considerations and Interactions

Milk thistle, known for its liver-protective qualities due to the active compound silymarin, necessitates careful consideration, particularly regarding its interactions with medications. Silymarin is a powerful antioxidant and anti-inflammatory agent, enhancing the liver's detoxification and regenerative capabilities. However, because it influences liver enzymes that metabolize drugs, milk thistle can alter the effectiveness of various medications, including drugs processed through the liver, such as painkillers, statins, diabetes medications, and anticoagulants, potentially leading to either increased side effects or reduced efficacy. Therefore, individuals taking prescription medications should consult with healthcare providers before starting milk thistle supplements to ensure no adverse interactions. Although milk thistle is generally safe, it should be used cautiously by those with a history of hormone-related cancers, as its effects on hormonal balance are not fully understood. Healthcare professionals advise pregnant or breast-feeding women to avoid milk thistle due to insufficient research on its safety in these groups. Thus, integrating milk thistle into a health regimen requires a balanced approach, weighing its benefits against potential risks and interactions to maintain overall health and safety.

For further reading, you can explore more details through the following link:

What Are The Benefits of Milk Thistle
https://www.verywellhealth.com/the-benefits-of-milk-thistle-88325

5.2 DANDELION ROOT: THE GENTLE DETOXIFIER FOR KIDNEYS AND LIVER

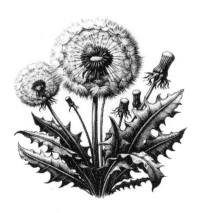

People often unjustly label dandelion root merely as a weed, yet it exhibits potent diuretic and detoxifying capabilities that are frequently underestimated. This often-ignored plant enhances the aesthetic diversity of gardens and offers profound health benefits, primarily through its root system. The roots of the dandelion are rich in compounds that actively support the purification processes of the liver and kidneys, organs essential to filtering and eliminating toxins from the body. These detoxification properties are particularly vital as they help maintain the body's overall well-being and resilience against illnesses by aiding in removing waste products. Furthermore, the dandelion root's ability to increase urine production naturally helps the body expel salts and excess water, thus further supporting the detox pathways. By incorporating dandelion root into diets or health regimens, individuals can leverage these natural properties to bolster their body's detoxification systems, showcasing the plant's value beyond its common perception.

Detoxifying Actions

Dandelion root is a natural diuretic; it fosters kidney function and promotes the elimination of waste and toxins through increased urine production. This gentle encouragement of the body's natural filtration system removes the absorbed toxic load, ensuring the kidneys operate efficiently and easily. Concurrently, the root's influence also extends to the liver, an organ besieged by the relentless task of neutralizing and expelling toxins. Dandelion Root stimulates bile flow, a crucial step in the digestive process that aids the liver in processing and purifying blood. Via this dual action—impacting both kidneys and liver—the plant orchestrates a comprehensive approach to detoxification.

Beyond its detoxifying prowess, dandelion root offers immunity-bolstering nutritional benefits, enhancing its role in health maintenance. Rich in vitamins A, C, and K, along with minerals such as potassium, iron, and zinc, the root nourishes the body at a cellular level. Inulin, a prebiotic fiber found in the root, further enriches this nourishing profile, fostering gut health and supporting the microbiome —two more allies in the body's defense against toxins.

Practical Applications

Incorporating dandelion root into a detox regimen can be a transformative practice deeply rooted in the popular tradition of tea rituals. This method involves simmering chopped dandelion root to create a decoction that infuses the water with its rich, earthy flavors and potent detoxifying properties. By engaging in this ritual regularly, the simple act of drinking tea transcends its usual purpose, becoming a daily purification ritual that honors the body's natural cleansing processes.

Making a dandelion root decoction is particularly effective because it allows for extracting a broad spectrum of healing compounds from the root. This process requires a longer simmering time than standard tea steeping, ensuring that the water releases the maximum amount of beneficial substances such as inulin, sesquiterpenes, and phenolic acids. The result is a concentrated liquid that individuals can dilute according to their taste preferences. It is a customizable and flexible option for those looking to harness the root's full detoxifying effects. This method provides a therapeutic level of dandelion root. It allows individuals to adjust the intensity and dosage of their detox tea, tailoring it to their specific health needs and detox goals. For those who need a more immediate way to enjoy dandelion, it is also available in capsule and tincture forms.

Considerations and interactions

While beneficial for detoxification, dandelion root's diuretic effect warrants caution among those on pharmaceutical diuretic medications, as the combined impact may lead to dehydration or electrolyte imbalances. Similarly, individuals on blood-thinning drugs must approach dandelion root with prudence, being mindful of its vitamin K content and corresponding potential to alter the effects of their medication. Ongoing dialogue and guidance from healthcare providers ensure that integrating dandelion roots into a health regimen enhances, rather than compromises, your health and well-being.

For further reading, you can explore more details through the following link:

11 Dandelion Root Benefits

What research says and what to consider before trying it
https://www.verywellhealth.com/the-benefits-of-dandelion-root-89103

5.3 CILANTRO AND TURMERIC: NATURAL CHELATORS FOR HEAVY METAL DETOX

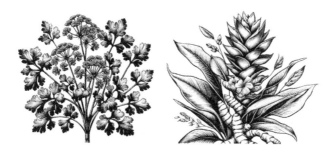

In the dynamic detoxification process, cilantro and turmeric play crucial, complementary roles. Cilantro, known for its chelating abilities, goes on the offense, actively assisting in removing heavy metals from the body, effectively pulling these toxins from tissues to aid in their elimination. Making cilantro a vital player in detoxification, particularly in combating heavy metal exposure. On the other hand, turmeric serves as a proactive protector of critical organs. Its active compound, curcumin, possesses potent anti-inflammatory and antioxidant properties, safeguarding organs against the potential damage from various toxins. Cilantro and Turmeric enhance the body's ability to cleanse and fortify itself against ongoing environmental and dietary assaults, orchestrating a holistic defense against toxicity. This partnership underscores the potent healing capabilities of these herbs in maintaining and enhancing organ health.

Detoxifying actions

Cilantro, with its delicate green leaves, serves not only as a culinary herb but also as an effective chelator, known for its ability to bind with and facilitate the removal of heavy metals like lead, mercury, and aluminum from the body. This action, derived from the Greek word 'chele,' meaning claw, highlights cilantro's potential to mitigate the toxic effects of these metals, a capability that limited yet promising empirical studies have supported. Complementing cilantro's detoxifying properties, turmeric, driven by its active compound curcumin, offers protective benefits, particularly for the liver, enhancing its ability to process and expel toxins—curcumin's anti-inflammatory properties further aid in reducing the bodily stresses associated with detoxification. Together, cilantro and turmeric form a potent detox duo, addressing the removal of existing toxins and the protection against new ones, representing a holistic approach to enhancing the body's natural detoxification processes.

Practical applications

As with other herbs, a successful strategy for integrating cilantro and turmeric into a detox regimen must be nuanced and requires paying due attention to dosage, preparation, and individual tolerance. Incorporating cilantro into the diet may begin with its regular direct inclusion in meals, from garnishes to green smoothies, ensuring a steady intake of its chelating properties. You can, however, be more versatile with turmeric's application; it can be consumed as a spice in culinary dishes or as a supplement in curcumin-extracted forms, offering flexibility in how one harnesses its benefits. The confluence of cilantro and turmeric in a detox diet amplifies the detoxification process. It enriches the body with nutrients and antioxidants, allowing you to nurture your body as you cleanse it. They come in capsule and tincture form if you are looking for other options.

Considerations and Interactions

Both scientific studies and anecdotal experiences point to cilantro and turmeric's effectiveness in heavy metal detoxification. While research provides a foundation for understanding the mechanisms through which these herbs act, anecdote testifies to a mosaic of outcomes, highlighting variability in individual responses and underscoring the imperativeness of approaching detoxification with an open yet discerning mind— recognizing that the rightful journey to purification is personal and multifaceted. Specific safety considerations regarding turmeric's influence on blood clotting and cilantro's potential to mobilize metals without adequate excretion necessitate a cautious approach. Consulting with health professionals ensures that the use of cilantro and turmeric aligns with one's health status and detox goals, crafting a pathway to detoxification that is both informed and intentional.

We looked at turmeric in chapter 3; for further reading on cilantro, you can explore more details through the following link:

Everything You Need to Know About Coriander (Cilantro)
https://www.verywellhealth.com/coriander-7488672

MAKE A DIFFERENCE WITH YOUR REVIEW
UNLOCK THE POWER OF GENEROSITY

"Helping one person might not change the whole world, but it could change the world for one person."

Imagine how rewarding it feels to share a *special secret* that makes someone's day better. That's the opportunity in front of us today, and I'm excited to invite you to be a part of it.

Would you *help* someone you've never met, even if you never got credit for it?

This person is a lot like you once were—curious about natural health, eager to learn about herbal remedies, and looking for *trusted* guidance.

Our mission is to make herbal medicine knowledge, like what's in *"Unlocking Wellness: Natural Herbal Remedies for Diseases"* by *Rami Archer,* accessible to everyone. Achieving this mission means reaching as many people as possible.

That's where you come in. Reviews are more than just feedback; they guide others who are seeking similar paths to wellness. Here's my ask on behalf of a reader you've never met:

Please consider leaving a review for this book.

It doesn't cost a penny and takes less than a minute, but your insights can profoundly impact someone else's journey to health and wellness.

Your review could help:

- *One more person avoid the side effects of synthetic medication.*
- *One more family use natural remedies to maintain their health.*
- *One more individual feel empowered about their health choices.*
- *One more reader reconnect with age-old wellness practices.*
- *One more story of healing and hope to begin.*

To share your thoughts and help a fellow seeker of natural health and wellness, just scan the QR code below or visit:

https://www.amazon.com/review/review-your-purchases/?asin=
B0DCGLTXJL

If you're ready to help someone discover the power of herbal remedies for diseases, then you are exactly who we love to support. Welcome to the community. You're one of us now!

I'm eager to help you explore more herbal secrets in the chapters ahead.

Thank you from the bottom of my heart for your generosity and support.

Your biggest fan, Rami Archer

PS - Remember, sharing valuable information increases your value in the eyes of others. If you think this book could help another, don't hesitate to pass it on!

CHAPTER 6
RESTORING HARMONY OF NOURISHMENT: HERBS FOR DIGESTIVE HEALTH

Maintaining digestive health plays a crucial yet understated role in our overall health and well-being in the intricate symphony of everyday life. Navigating the complexities of daily life, where irregular meal times and quick eating habits are all too common, can often lead to digestive imbalances. Fighting these imbalances is where the natural potency of specific herbs steps into the spotlight, offering a melody of relief and support. Peppermint, for instance, is not just a refreshing flavor—it is a powerful aid in alleviating symptoms associated with Irritable Bowel Syndrome (IBS) and soothing general digestive discomfort. Similarly, ginger is a versatile remedy, effectively calming nausea and aiding digestion.

Additionally, fennel seeds are a traditional go-to for their carminative properties, helping to ease bloating and gas. At the same time, chamomile and gentian roots provide gentle support for overall stomach health and digestive harmony. Together, these herbs create a chorus of solutions that restore balance to our digestive systems, ensuring that they meet our body's nutritional needs in harmony despite the chaos of our routines. This holistic approach improves digestion and enhances our absorption of nutrients, promoting a healthier, more balanced lifestyle.

6.1 PEPPERMINT: SOOTHING DIGESTIVE DISCOMFORT AND IBS

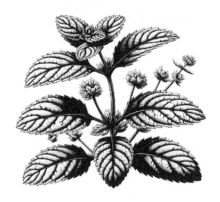

Peppermint is renowned for its cool, refreshing properties and plays a crucial role in soothing the digestive system and alleviating discomfort associated with various gastrointestinal issues. The natural compounds in peppermint leaves, particularly menthol, relax the gastrointestinal tract's smooth muscles, which helps reduce the muscle spasms commonly associated with irritable bowel syndrome (IBS) and other digestive disorders. This action not only eases symptoms such as abdominal pain, bloating, and irregular bowel movements but also improves overall digestive health. Furthermore, the cooling sensation of peppermint aids in reducing inflammation within the gastrointestinal tract, enhancing comfort and promoting healing. Given its antispasmodic properties and ability to improve digestive motility, health experts often recommend peppermint as a natural and effective treatment. It is available in various forms, including dietary supplements like capsules and extracts and traditional herbal teas, offering a gentle, accessible alternative to pharmaceutical options for those seeking to enhance their digestive wellness naturally.

Practical Applications

Incorporating peppermint into your daily routine offers a straightforward and effective way to enhance digestive health and overall well-being. One of the most popular and enjoyable methods is starting the day with a hot cup of peppermint tea. To prepare, steep dried peppermint leaves in boiling water for five to ten minutes; this method allows the menthol and other beneficial compounds to infuse the water, maximizing the tea's soothing properties. The aromatic vapor can calm the digestive system even before the first sip, making it a perfect, tranquil way to start the morning or unwind between meals. Peppermint oil capsules provide a practical alternative for those seeking a more potent or convenient intake form. These capsules deliver a precise dose of menthol, ensuring consistent digestive relief and fitting seamlessly into even the busiest schedules. Additionally, peppermint tinctures offer another versatile option; they can be added to water or tea for a quick and effective remedy, providing flexibility in dosage and use. Regular use of peppermint, whether as tea, capsules, or tinctures, not only aids digestion but also integrates moments of calm into daily life, supporting a holistic approach to health and wellness.

Considerations and Interactions

Peppermint, renowned for its soothing properties for those with Irritable Bowel Syndrome (IBS), can paradoxically pose challenges for individuals with gastroesophageal reflux disease (GERD). The herb's ability to relax the lower esophageal sphincter, while beneficial in reducing intestinal spasms associated with IBS, can exacerbate GERD symptoms by enabling stomach acids to flow back into the esophagus more freely. Underscoring the nuanced approach required when using herbal remedies, as their effects can vary significantly based on individual health conditions.

Understanding and navigating these contraindications is crucial for safely integrating herbs like peppermint into a health regimen. This situation exemplifies why it's essential to tailor herbal treatments to individual health profiles, ensuring that the selected remedy supports overall health without causing unintended harm. Health-care providers often recommend that patients with GERD avoid peppermint to prevent the aggravation of their condition, high-lighting the importance of personalized medical advice when considering herbal remedies. This customized approach ensures that each individual receives the most benefit from their treatments while minimizing potential risks.

For further reading, you can explore more details through the following link:

What to Know About the Benefits of Peppermint Leaf
https://www.verywellhealth.com/peppermint-uses-dosage-and-more-7511339

6.2 GINGER: A VERSATILE REMEDY FOR NAUSEA AND INDIGESTION

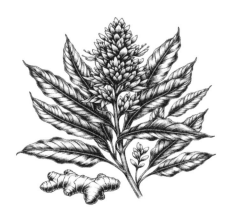

Ginger is widely celebrated for its robust flavor and health benefits, especially its effectiveness in alleviating nausea. Revered across various cultures, ginger's piquant aroma and fiery taste make it a preferred remedy for those experiencing motion or morning sickness during pregnancy. The root's natural compounds interact with the body to soothe the stomach and calm the digestive system, making it a trusted component in the arsenal of herbal medicine.

This traditional use of ginger extends beyond mere folklore, as it has become a cornerstone in herbal practices for its reliable anti-nausea properties. Whether consumed as a fresh root, steeped in tea or as a supplement, ginger provides significant relief for those afflicted by the discomfort of nausea. Its ability to mitigate these symptoms without causing harm makes it particularly valuable for pregnant women seeking natural remedies to ease morning sickness, further solidifying its status as a beacon of relief in natural health care.

Digestive Actions

Ginger root, celebrated in traditional and modern medicine, is highly effective in alleviating nausea due to its bioactive compounds, gingerol, and shogaol. These compounds interact with the digestive and central nervous systems by modulating serotonergic receptors and enhancing gastrointestinal function, effectively reducing the urge to vomit. This interaction makes ginger particularly beneficial for those prone to motion sickness on sea voyages or women experiencing morning sickness during pregnancy, offering a natural alternative to pharmaceuticals without sedative side effects. Beyond its anti-nausea properties, ginger also acts as a digestive stimulant, enhancing the digestive process by stimulating enzyme secretion and improving gut motility. This comprehensive action alleviates symptoms of indigestion and promotes overall digestive health, ensuring efficient nutrient breakdown and absorption and supporting the body's ability to derive maximum nourishment from food.

Practical Applications

Ginger's ready versatility of culinary and medicinal applications allows for its seamless integration into daily dietary practices. Simmered in boiling water, a slice of fresh ginger morphs into a tea that warms the body and soothes the stomach. This simple preparation, accessible to anyone with a kettle and a few minutes to spare, is a quick remedy for nausea and an effective pre-meal digestive aid. If you seek ginger's benefits without the kick of its spicy flavor, capsules containing ginger extract provide a concentrated dose of its active compounds, offering convenience and potency in equal measure. Culinary explorations further expand ginger's repertoire of availability—from the zest it lends to stir-fries and soups to the refreshing tang of ginger-infused beverages—making its inclusion in healthful and flavorful meals.

Considerations and Interactions

Alongside these meaningful benefits, ginger's broader safety profile is more nuanced. While ginger's anticoagulant properties are mild compared to its pharmaceutical blood-thinning counterparts, it does have the potential to interact with blood-thinning medications, necessitating caution and, ideally, consultation with a healthcare provider to ensure its incorporation into your regimen complements existing treatments while avoiding unintended complications.

While widespread use and research affirming its safety underscore ginger's endorsement as a remedy to assuage the effects of morning sickness, pregnancy nonetheless invites an exceedingly measured approach. Pregnant women, guided by their health practitioners, might find ginger a gentle, effective remedy, but the principles of moderation and oversight remain paramount for safeguarding both mother and child.

We explored ginger earlier, refer back to chapter 1.

6.3 FENNEL: REDUCING BLOATING AND GAS NATURALLY

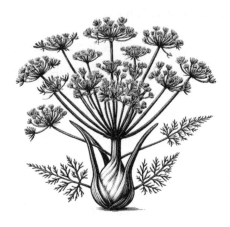

With its rich history rooted in ancient medicinal practices, fennel is a natural remedy for common digestive issues such as bloating and gas. Esteemed in Greek and Roman cultures, people appreciate this herb for its unique anise-like flavor and digestive benefits. Fennel's effectiveness in calming the stomach and easing digestion is due primarily to its active compound, anethole, which has antispasmodic and anti-inflammatory properties. These properties help to relax the gastrointestinal tract's smooth muscles, reducing spasms that contribute to gas and bloating, thereby promoting a smoother digestive process.

Regularly using fennel in diet or as an herbal tea can significantly enhance digestive wellness. It offers a gentle yet potent solution to discomfort, making fennel a beloved component of natural health regimens, particularly in holistic and traditional medicine, where gentle and natural remedies are preferred. Its holistic impact on digestive health alleviates immediate symptoms and contributes to long-term gastrointestinal function, reinforcing fennel's role as a vital digestive aid in herbal medicine circles.

Digestive Actions

Fennel, known for its carminative properties derived from the Latin term 'carminare,' meaning 'to card wool,' effectively eases gastrointestinal discomfort by releasing trapped gas, alleviating bloating and pressure. The seeds of the fennel plant act as a soothing balm for the digestive tract's lining, calming the discomfort often associated with digestion. Anethole is at the core of fennel's therapeutic effects, a compound responsible for its distinctive sweet, anise-like aroma. Anethole is crucial in soothing the digestive system and potentially reducing inflammation, allowing for smoother digestion with minimal disruption. It triggers a series of bodily responses that relieve spasms, promote the expulsion of gas, and improve overall digestive harmony, thereby enhancing the efficiency and comfort of the digestive process. Through these mechanisms, fennel supports a balanced and effective digestive system, making it a valuable natural remedy for various digestive ailments.

Practical Applications

Incorporating fennel seeds into your dietary regimen offers numerous ways to harness their digestive benefits, ranging from quick relief methods to more gradual, sustained approaches. For swift alleviation of bloating and gas, chewing a small spoonful of raw fennel seeds releases their essential oils directly into the digestive system, providing immediate relief. While subject to individual needs, the recommended dosage typically aligns with moderation, underscoring the wisdom of balance in herbal remedies. On the other hand, brewing a warm tea from crushed fennel seeds utilizes their carminative properties to soothe the digestive tract. It serves as a ritual that enhances holistic health and well-being. This tea preparation process invites a moment of calm and mindfulness into your daily routine, reinforcing the holistic benefits of fennel beyond mere physical digestion.

Moreover, for those who prefer incorporating the benefits of fennel more subtly, adding ground fennel seeds to foods like salads, dressings, or homemade breads ensures a continuous intake of their beneficial properties throughout the day. This method allows the digestive advantages of fennel to be seamlessly integrated into meals, making the use of this herb both effective and enjoyable. As these seeds become part of regular meals, they support digestive health and contribute to a balanced approach to dietary habits, promoting overall well-being through the natural power of herbal remedies.

Considerations and Interactions

While fennel's benefits paint a picture of digestive ease, certain precautions warrant attention. Although rare, allergic reactions necessitate a mindful introduction of fennel seeds into the diet, especially among those with sensitivities to plants in the Apiaceae family. This vigilance ensures that the path to digestive comfort is paved with caution, respecting the body's signals and responses. Furthermore, interactions with certain medications—particularly those affecting blood clotting or hormone-sensitive conditions— underscore the importance of consulting with a healthcare provider before embracing fennel as a digestive remedy.

For further reading, you can explore more details through the following link:

Fennel and Fennel Seeds: Look at the Benefits
https://www.verywellhealth.com/fennel-and-fennel-seeds-benefits-uses-and-more-7495392

6.4 CHAMOMILE AND GENTIAN: GENTLE HERBS FOR STOMACH HEALTH, DIGESTIVE SUPPORT

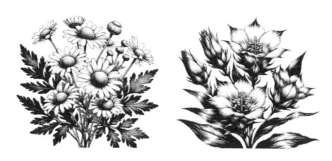

Chamomile and gentian are revered herbs in traditional medicine, each playing a critical role in supporting digestive health. Chamomile is celebrated for its anti-inflammatory and soothing properties, making it highly effective in alleviating gastrointestinal discomfort such as bloating and abdominal cramps. Its calming influence extends throughout the digestive tract, enhancing gut health and facilitating smoother digestive processes, relieving immediate discomfort and promoting long-term digestive wellness. Conversely, gentian serves as a powerful digestive stimulant, improving the secretion of digestive enzymes essential for the effective breakdown and absorption of nutrients, thereby optimizing gastrointestinal efficiency. When used together, chamomile and gentian offer a comprehensive approach to digestive health; chamomile's soothing effects complement gentian's stimulating properties, creating a balanced digestive aid strategy that supports overall gut health and function, embodying a holistic method to maintain gastrointestinal wellness.

Digestive Actions

Chamomile and gentian root are invaluable herbs in enhancing digestive wellness, each supported by both traditional use and scientific research. Chamomile's essential oils soothe the stomach lining, easing discomfort and promoting relaxation of the nervous system, which not only alleviates immediate digestive disturbances but also supports immune health and reduces inflammation, contributing to long-term digestive health. Regular consumption of chamomile tea is particularly beneficial for managing symptoms of chronic digestive conditions. On the other hand, people celebrate gentian root for its digestive-stimulating effects, as its bitter compounds activate the body's digestive enzymes for more efficient nutrient breakdown and assimilation. This activation improves metabolism and boosts energy levels while supporting liver function and stimulating appetite, which is especially beneficial for those with sluggish digestive systems. Chamomile and gentian offer a synergistic approach that calms and enhances the digestive system, providing robust support that addresses various digestive challenges, from minor discomforts to more severe conditions, fostering comprehensive digestive health.

Practical applications

A digestive tonic can harness the alliance of chamomile's calming properties —to temper your stomach's distress—and gentian's capacity for stimulation—to invigorate digestive processes that may have languished in inertia. Preparing such a tonic involves blending teas or tinctures from these herbs, a deliberate act of self-care that, in turn, nurtures the digestive system back to a state of optimal function. The guiding principle in this kind of synergistic application lies in the delicate art of dosing. Tonic proportions of both chamomile and gentian must be tailored to individual digestive profiles, ensuring a therapeutic effect that is both potent and harmonious.

Alternatively, brewing a tea combining chamomile flowers and gentian root can be practical and enjoyable. This method allows the water to extract the soluble compounds from the herbs into a therapeutic elixir. You can customize the ratio of herbs based on your taste preferences and tolerance, starting with a milder quantity of gentian to ease into its strong bitterness. For more targeted support, tinctures offer a concentrated form of the herbs' benefits, allowing for precise dosing with the advice of a holistic health practitioner. This method ensures that the dosage respects your body's limits while optimizing the therapeutic effects.

Considerations and Interactions

While chamomile and gentian are revered for their digestive health benefits, it is crucial to consider potential contraindications and individual health backgrounds when using these herbs. Gentian, known for its stimulating effects on the digestive system, may not be suitable for individuals with gallbladder issues or acute gastrointestinal inflammation as it could exacerbate their condition. Similarly, chamomile, typically safe and effective, may pose risks for those allergic to the Asteraceae family, potentially triggering allergic reactions. The therapeutic use of chamomile and gentian highlights their role in holistic wellness practices, emphasizing the importance of addressing the whole person—body, mind, and spirit —and reflecting an understanding of the interconnectedness of human health. As the exploration of herbal medicine continues to expand, leveraging the earth's bounty for health solutions, it enhances our appreciation for the rich tapestry of plant-based healing developed over centuries. This journey into herbal medicine not only deepens our understanding of natural health but also teaches us to utilize nature's intrinsic capabilities to nurture and sustain our well-being, all while embracing the wisdom of traditional medicinal practices:

For further reading, you can explore more details through the following links:

GERMAN CHAMOMILE: Uses, Safety

https://www.verywellhealth.com/the-benefits-of-chamomile-89436

Gentian

https://www.drugs.com/npp/gentian.html

CHAPTER 7

FORTIFYING THE BASTIONS OF HEALTH: HERBAL ALLIES IN IMMUNE SUPPORT

E nhancing our immune system is critical to safeguarding our well-being in the relentless pursuit of robust health. Among nature's abundant resources, a cadre of herbs distinctly stands out for their immune-boosting capabilities, drawing from centuries of traditional medicinal practices. At the forefront, echinacea is celebrated for its effectiveness in enhancing immune responses, making it a go-to remedy in herbal immune support circles. Alongside, astragalus acts not merely as a supplement but as a stalwart defender, fortifying the body's resilience against bacterial and viral invaders.

Elderberry joins this elite group with its rich antiviral properties and high antioxidant content, helping prevent illness onset and speed recovery. Equally formidable is Garlic, revered as a natural antibiotic; its widespread use in various cultures underscores its potent effects in fighting infections. Further enriching this herbal repertoire, andrographis and cat's claw stand out for their robust anti-inflammatory and infection-fighting abilities. Together, these herbs form a formidable line of defense, offering a natural, holistic approach to maintaining health and preventing disease, thus embodying the essence of preventive healthcare.

7.1 ECHINACEA: NATURE'S IMMUNE BOOSTER

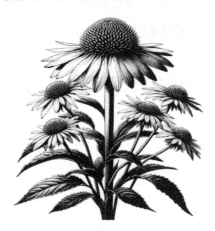

In the vast and varied world of natural health remedies, echinacea holds a place of honor. Amid the complex challenges of human health, this powerful herb emerges as a beacon of fortification, standing firm as nature's answer to boosting our immune defenses. Its rich history in traditional medicine spans centuries, with countless individuals relying on its efficacy to enhance bodily resilience against common ailments. Echinacea's role extends beyond mere symptom relief; it actively strengthens the immune system, preparing the body to ward off and fight infections more effectively.

Echinacea is known for stimulating the production of immune cells and increasing the body's response to microbial invaders. In an era when health is increasingly fragile, echinacea offers a natural, proactive approach to health maintenance. By integrating this herb into our wellness routines, we embrace a holistic strategy that aligns with the rhythms of nature, ensuring a more robust existence and a fortified defense against the health challenges of modern life.

Immunization Actions

Echinacea, named after the Greek word 'echinos, which means hedgehog, aptly describes its role in bolstering the immune system, much like the spiny defense of a hedgehog. This herb enhances the body's immune response, activates the production of white blood cells, and improves the functionality of the lymphatic system.

Primarily used to combat common respiratory ailments such as the common cold and influenza, echinacea does not directly attack the responsible viruses but strengthens the body's defenses. By enhancing the immune system, echinacea helps prevent infections from gaining a foothold and slows their progression if they penetrate the body's initial barriers. This enhancement makes echinacea an essential tool for preventive health during the peak seasons of colds and flu, helping individuals not only stave off illness but also recover more swiftly from symptoms, thereby maintaining better overall health.

Practical Applications

Echinacea's versatility in form—tincture, tea, and capsule—makes it a flexible option for enhancing immune health. For those seeking swift immune support at the onset of cold and flu season, echinacea tincture is a practical choice. Typically administered in small doses, about 2-4 ml taken three times a day, its concentrated extracts offer rapid absorption and immediate action. During the colder months, echinacea tea provides a comforting alternative, combining a hot beverage's soothing warmth with the herb's immune-boosting properties. Enjoying 1-2 cups daily can enhance your body's defenses while providing a calming ritual. Capsules, offering a more controlled dosage, are ideal for consistent supplementation; a standard recommendation is one to two 300-500 mg capsules taken with meals, up to three times per day during active cold and flu periods. Regardless of the form chosen, adhering to these recommended dosages maximizes the immune-stimulating benefits of echinacea while maintaining safety and efficacy.

Considerations and Interactions

When considering echinacea for its immune-boosting benefits, it's essential to be aware of its potential interactions and the necessary safety precautions. Particularly for individuals with autoimmune disorders, the stimulatory effects of echinacea on the immune system can exacerbate symptoms or interfere with the condition's management. Additionally, those on immunosuppressive medications should exercise caution, as echinacea might counteract the intended effects of these drugs, diminishing their efficacy. It is also essential to consider echinacea's interactions with other pharmaceuticals, as it may alter the effectiveness of certain medications, including some metabolized by the liver. Given these considerations, anyone contemplating the use of echinacea should first consult with healthcare professionals. This dialogue ensures that echinacea is incorporated into one's health regimen safely and effectively, enhancing overall well-being without unintended consequences.

For further reading, you can explore more details through the following link:

Echinacea: Everything You Need to Know
https://www.verywellhealth.com/echinacea-benefits-side-effects-and-more-7503379

7.2 ASTRAGALUS: THE PROTECTOR HERB

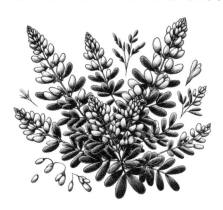

Astragalus, a revered herb in traditional Chinese medicine, has been used for centuries to enhance protective health. This powerful adaptogen is known for fortifying the body's immune system, effectively creating a formidable barrier against microbial invasions. The primary mechanism through which astragalus operates is by boosting the production of white blood cells, the body's main line of defense against infectious agents. This increase in white blood cells is critical for combating pathogens and warding off infections.

Furthermore, astragalus enhances the body's resilience to biological pathogens and physical and emotional stress, improving the immune response. Its ability to modulate the body's stress response and strengthen immune function makes it particularly valuable when the immune system might be compromised, such as during seasonal transitions or stressful periods. The herb's broad-spectrum benefits extend beyond mere disease prevention; astragalus also helps maintain the body's energy levels and supports various metabolic processes, ensuring that the body can sustain its defenses against the continual challenges posed by pathogens in our environment.

Immunization Actions

Astragalus (Astragalus membranaceus) goes beyond bolstering the body's immune response. It profoundly reinforces the body's inherent mechanisms of resilience, enabling a fortified stance against the onslaught of infections.

The herb operates subtly over time to erect a fortified barrier against pathogenic attacks on the body. Astragalus achieves this effect through multifaceted immune engagement, stimulating the activity of macrophages (voracious cells that devour pathogens) and enhancing the production of T-cells (the orchestrators of the immune response). This vigilant, robust defense actively maintains a dynamic equilibrium, swiftly and steadily responding to the threat of infection.

The astragalus uses its flavonoid and saponin compounds to neutralize antioxidant defense on the cellular level. It mitigates the radicals' potential for harm and preserves the immune system's functional vitality by ensuring its mechanisms remain unimpeded by oxidative damage.

Practical Applications

Integrating astragalus into daily health regimens involves a strategic approach that harmonizes with your lifestyle and a broader scope of health and wellness practices and objectives. For those inclined towards the culinary arts, you can ingest it via dietary sources, as the root's subtly sweet flavor expresses nicely in soups and broths; consider adding its root to slow-cooked dishes to achieve a particular depth of flavor. You can also ingest it in supplement forms, such as capsules and tinctures that concentrate its properties for ease of use. Still, you must choose these products judiciously, prioritizing quality and purity. This holistic approach to incorporating astragalus, attuned to the nuances of individual health goals and preferences, embodies a comprehensive strategy for immune support that leverages the herb's potential to foster resilience and vitality.

Considerations and Interactions

Astragalus (Astragalus membranaceus), a traditional herbal remedy, is valued for its immune-boosting and antioxidant properties but requires careful usage to ensure safety and efficacy. Mainly, individuals with autoimmune diseases should use astragalus with caution due to its potential to stimulate an already overactive immune system, possibly worsening symptoms. Furthermore, astragalus can interfere with immunosuppressive medications by counteracting their effects, and it may alter the efficacy or safety of other drugs metabolized by the liver's cytochrome P450 enzyme system. Those on anticoagulant therapy should know astragalus's blood-thinning properties, which could heighten bleeding risks. Additionally, its diuretic properties might increase dehydration and electrolyte imbalances when combined with other diuretics. Therefore, it is crucial for anyone considering astragalus, especially those with pre-existing conditions or those taking other medications, to consult healthcare providers to tailor a treatment plan that maximizes benefits while mitigating risks.

For further reading, you can explore more details through the following link:

What is Astragalus Good For?
https://www.verywellhealth.com/astragalus-what-should-i-know-about-it-89410

7.3 ELDERBERRY: THE ANTIVIRAL SUPERFRUIT

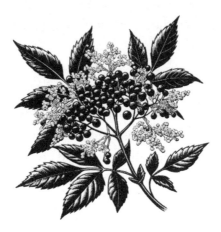

Elderberry, the Sambucus tree's fruit, is a testament to nature's remarkable simplicity and medicinal potency. Throughout the ages, this small, dark berry has been revered in folk medicine, woven into the fabric of cultural health practices for its immune-boosting properties. As a harbinger of immune fortification, elderberry is celebrated not only for its rich nutritional profile—abundant in vitamins and antioxidants—but also for its efficacy in the fight against viral infections, particularly influenza. The active compounds in elderberries, such as anthocyanins, are recognized for their antioxidant properties and ability to enhance the body's immune response significantly. These properties help to shorten the duration and reduce the severity of flu symptoms, making elderberry a formidable opponent against viral foes. Vitamins and nutrients that contribute to their health benefits. Some of the critical vitamins found in elderberries include:

- **1. Vitamin C**
- **2. Vitamin A**
- **3. Vitamins B1 (Thiamine)**
- **4. Vitamins B2 (Riboflavin)**
- **5. Vitamins B6**

These vitamins and other nutrients, such as dietary fiber, antioxidants, and flavonoids, make elderberries a highly beneficial addition to a health-focused diet, particularly for enhancing immune function.

Immunization Actions

Elderberry modulates the immune response via a delicate calibration and enhancement of the body's defenses. Specifically, it stimulates cytokine production, a protein crucial to the immune system's communication network, thus ensuring a coordinated and robust bodily response to infections—delicately modulating and optimizing defense mechanisms without tipping into overstimulation. The result is a fortified, resilient, vigilant immune landscape, ready to confront pathogenic challenges with renewed vigor.

Practical Applications

Elderberry syrup and tea are practical applications of elderberries that harness their antiviral and immune-boosting properties through different preparation methods. Simmering elderberries creates elderberry syrup in water to extract their essential nutrients, particularly anthocyanins, and other antioxidants, which are pivotal in combating viral infections like the flu. After simmering, strain the mixture to remove berry solids. Add natural sweeteners like honey or maple syrup to enhance flavor and boost medicinal qualities by soothing the throat and supporting the immune system. This syrup can be taken at the onset of flu symptoms or regularly during flu season as a preventive measure. Alternatively, elderberry tea is made by steeping dried elderberries in boiling water to create a therapeutic beverage, often with additional immune-supporting herbs like echinacea or ginger. This steeping process infuses the water with nutrients from the elderberries, resulting in a healing, comforting tea ideal for cold weather or when feeling unwell, embodying a nurturing self-care practice that promotes health with every sip. You can also find elderberries' immune-boosting properties in capsule and tincture form.

Considerations and Interactions

Effectively harnessing the benefits of elderberry requires meticulous attention to its potent properties, including proper identification and preparation to avoid potential risks. The plant's leaves, stems, and unripe berries contain glycosides that can release cyanogenic compounds, potentially leading to cyanide exposure. To ensure safety, it is crucial to thoroughly cook or process elderberries to deactivate these harmful compounds and source them from reputable suppliers who adhere to safe preparation practices. Although typically safe for most individuals, elderberry should be avoided by those with autoimmune diseases due to its immune-stimulating effects, and pregnant or breastfeeding women should consult healthcare providers before use. Elderberry's antiviral efficacy and immune-modulating capabilities make it a valuable natural remedy. Still, users must handle it responsibly and cautiously to safely and effectively tap into its full health-enhancing potential.

For further reading, you can explore more details through the following link:

What is Elderberry Good For?

https://www.verywellhealth.com/elderberry-for-colds-and-flu-can-it-help-89559

7.4 GARLIC: THE NATURAL ANTIBIOTIC

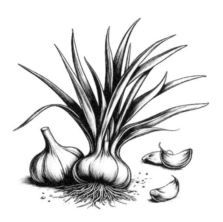

Garlic, scientifically known as Allium sativum, is celebrated in both culinary and medicinal contexts for its potent antibacterial and antiviral properties. When you crush or chop garlic cloves, they release their primary active component, allicin, initiating a chemical reaction that produces this sulfur-containing compound that is effective in combating various pathogens. This natural antibiotic disrupts the cellular structures of pathogens, hindering their ability to reproduce and establishing garlic as a formidable antimicrobial agent. Beyond fighting infections, garlic boosts the immune system, reduces blood pressure, and aids cardiovascular health, solidifying its role as a broad-spectrum therapeutic agent. Its enduring use across different cultures and centuries highlights its significant contribution to traditional and contemporary medical practices, making garlic a vital and timeless remedy in the global fight against illness.

Immunization Actions

Garlic, scientifically known as Allium sativum, is renowned for its potent antimicrobial properties, derived primarily from its cloves. When garlic cloves are crushed or chopped, they undergo a chemical reaction that releases allicin, a powerful compound that acts as a significant disruptor of pathogenic defenses. This transformation allows the garlic to effectively attack and break down the defenses of various pathogens, enhancing its capability to combat a broad spectrum of microbial threats. Allicin's ability to interfere with the life cycles and reproductive mechanisms of bacteria and viruses makes garlic an effective natural remedy against respiratory and gastrointestinal infections. Its use extends beyond the kitchen; people also use it medicinally to boost the body's defenses, making it an integral part of preventive health practices. Garlic's role as a natural antibiotic has been revered in traditional and modern health strategies, making it a crucial element in combating diseases ranging from the common cold to more severe bacterial infections.

Additional Circulatory Actions

Garlic significantly contributes to cardiovascular health by improving circulatory system functions through its bioactive compounds. These compounds enhance the bioavailability of nitric oxide, a critical vasodilation agent that relaxes and expands blood vessels, thereby lowering systemic blood pressure and reducing the workload on the heart. This mechanism is essential for preventing hypertension and diminishing the risk of heart disease. Additionally, garlic is crucial in lipid management because it influences lipid profiles to lower serum cholesterol levels. This reduction is vital for decreasing the buildup of arterial plaques, which are precursors to more serious cardiovascular conditions such as arteriosclerosis. By helping to prevent plaque accumulation, garlic supports arterial health and reduces the risk of heart attacks and strokes. Its dual action of enhancing vascular function and managing cholesterol levels makes garlic a powerful natural ally in combating cardiovascular diseases and a valuable addition to a heart-healthy diet.

Practical Applications

Incorporating garlic into daily diets enhances the flavor of meals and bridges culinary pleasure and medicinal benefits, particularly for immune and cardiovascular health. Consuming raw garlic cloves is the most effective way to harness the high levels of allicin, garlic's most potent bioactive compound, known for its intense flavor and significant health properties. However, the sharp pungency of raw garlic may be overwhelming for some, prompting culinary enthusiasts to explore alternative methods such as cooking. While cooking garlic reduces its allicin content, it still contributes health benefits by transforming its sharp flavor into a savory depth that complements a variety of dishes like sauces, soups, stir-fries, and marinades. For those opposed to the strong taste of raw or cooked garlic, supplements provide:

- *A convenient alternative.*
- *Encapsulating garlic's active compounds such as allicin and alliin.*
- *Thus offering a balance between convenience and health efficacy.*

Whether one chooses the robust intensity of raw garlic, the mellower taste of cooked garlic, or the neutral option of supplements, integrating garlic into daily routines can significantly bolster immune function and cardiovascular health, adapting its vast potential to individual health needs and dietary preferences.

Considerations and Interactions

Garlic is renowned for its health benefits, but it also poses some risks, particularly regarding digestive health and interactions with certain medications. After consuming garlic, some individuals may experience digestive discomfort, such as bloating, gas, or an upset stomach. This discomfort is generally transient but unpleasant, highlighting the need for moderation and thoughtful integration of garlic into the diet. Those affected may benefit from reducing the amount of garlic consumed or gradually incorporating it into their meals to minimize adverse effects. Moreover, garlic's ability to affect blood clotting mechanisms can enhance the effects of anticoagulant medications like warfarin, increasing the risk of bleeding. This interaction necessitates caution and professional healthcare guidance for those taking such drugs. Consulting with healthcare providers before integrating garlic into a dietary regimen can ensure its benefits—particularly cardiovascular health—are realized safely and effectively without compromising overall health through negative medication interactions.

For further reading on garlic, refer back to chapter 1.

7.5 ANDROGRAPHIS AND CAT'S CLAW: HERBAL WARRIORS AGAINST INFECTION

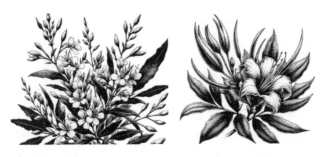

Andrographis and cat's claw are distinguished botanical warriors in herbal medicine, renowned for their ability to combat respiratory infections effectively. Andrographis, known as the "King of Bitters," showcases potent anti-inflammatory and antiviral properties that make it highly effective against respiratory pathogens like cold and flu viruses. Its active compounds, andrographolides, enhance immune system activity and significantly reduce the severity and duration of symptoms, making it a popular choice during the cold and flu season. On the other hand, cat's claw, sourced from a vine native to the Amazon rainforest, is celebrated for its immune-stimulating and anti-inflammatory effects. It contains unique alkaloids that boost white blood cell response and inhibit viral replication, providing a comprehensive defense mechanism against infections. Andrographis and cat's claw form a formidable duo, bolstering the body's defenses and offering a holistic approach to managing and preventing respiratory ailments, symbolizing resilience and hope in the ongoing battle against microbial threats.

Immunization Actions

Andrographis and cat's claw are potent herbs that synergistically combat respiratory infections through anti-inflammatory and immune-stimulating properties. Andrographis contains andrographolide, a critical compound that interacts with cellular signaling pathways to reduce the release of cytokines, thereby alleviating inflammation and discomfort associated with respiratory ailments and speeding up recovery. Concurrently, cat's claw, distinguished by its curved thorns, is rich in alkaloids and phytochemicals that enhance the immune system's ability to fight infections. It explicitly boosts phagocytosis, where immune cells engulf and neutralize pathogens. Additionally, its anti-inflammatory properties ensure a balanced immune response, preventing excessive inflammation that can complicate infections. Together, andrographis and cat's claw offer a holistic approach to managing respiratory health, embodying the principle that the combined effects of these herbs are more significant than their individual contributions, effectively preventing and mitigating respiratory infections.

Practical Applications

Andrographis and cat's claw are highly effective in combating respiratory infections, making them essential during the cold and flu season. Andrographis can be taken in various forms, such as teas, tinctures, or capsules, each providing a convenient method to harness its benefits. The active compounds, andrographolides, are primarily known for boosting the immune system and reducing the duration and severity of symptoms.

On the other hand, cat's claw supports immune function with its unique alkaloids that enhance white blood cell response and inhibit viral replication. Cat's Claw is available in similar formats—teas, which offer a soothing way to absorb its benefits; tinctures, which provide concentrated doses; and capsules, perfect for those seeking a quick and direct method of consumption. Utilizing andrographis and cat's claw in these forms can significantly aid in preventing and alleviating respiratory ailments, offering a holistic approach to health during peak infection times.

Considerations and Interactions

The potent nature of andrographis and cat's claw necessitates a mindful approach to their use, particularly among individuals navigating the complexities of autoimmune conditions or those under the regimen of immunosuppressive medications. While beneficial in infection prevention and treatment, the immune-stimulating effects of these herbs may pose challenges and risks to conditions marked by an overly active immune response. As such, professional health-care guidance is necessary to ensure the incorporation of andrographis and cat's claw into holistic health practices is safe and appropriate.

Andrographis and cat's claw's respective roles in combating respiratory infections and fortifying the body's defenses illuminate the potential for natural remedies to act not as mere supplements but as integral components of a holistic team approach to health and well-being.

The complex interplay of botanical properties, immune responses, and health practices enriches our understanding of the body's resilience and the role of nature in nurturing this innate strength. A deepened understanding of herbal wisdom's relationship to and impact on immunity and infection, in turn, deepens our appreciation for the intricate dance of health and disease, one guided by the timeless rhythm of nature's remedies.

For further reading, you can explore more details through the following links:

Andrographis
https://www.drugs.com/npp/andrographis.html

Cat's Claw: A Traditional Herbal Remedy That Should Be Used With Caution
https://www.verywellhealth.com/cats-claw-benefits-and-safety-8379773

CHAPTER 8
CULTIVATING EQUILIBRIUM: ADAPTOGENS IN STRESS ALLEVIATION

In the tumult of modern life, where the relentless pace can overwhelm our mental and physical health and wellness, nature offers a timeless solution in the form of adaptogens. These remarkable botanicals, such as ashwagandha, holy basil, chamomile, lavender, rhodiola, and ginseng, have been used for centuries to manage stress and enhance balance. Adaptogens modulate the body's stress response systems, providing stability and resilience in the face of daily pressures. They act as natural guardians, harmonizing the dynamic interplay between humans and their environments, enabling individuals to navigate life's challenges with greater ease and stability.

Adaptogens achieve their effects by fine-tuning the endocrine and nervous systems, ensuring the body can maintain homeostasis despite fluctuating external conditions. This capability allows individuals to weave resilience into their daily routines, stepping back from the brink of exhaustion to reclaim moments of calm and clarity. In integrating these potent herbs into everyday life, we tap into a profound source of natural health that empowers us to manage stress more effectively and sustain our overall well-being. The enduring relevance of adaptogens in our quest for wellness highlights a fundamental truth: often, the solutions we seek are embedded in the natural world around us, waiting to be rediscovered and embraced as essential elements of a balanced life.

Stress-Modulating Actions

Adaptogens, introduced by Soviet scientist N.V. Lazarev in 1947, represent a unique class of botanicals, including herbs and mushrooms, known for supporting the body's ability to manage stress, fatigue, and anxiety. These natural agents act as biological response modifiers, enhancing resilience to various physical, chemical, and biological stressors and promoting homeostasis without the harsh impacts of stimulants. Instead of triggering an intense response, adaptogens subtly encourage the body towards equilibrium, moderating the stress response to maintain optimal functionality. This action is invaluable in today's world, where stress is pervasive and complex, helping to sustain mental and physical performance under pressure, boost stamina against fatigue, stabilize mood amidst anxiety, and prevent burnout. Moreover, adaptogens offer holistic benefits by bolstering the immune system, protecting against oxidative stress, and enhancing overall vitality, making them essential for anyone seeking to improve health and cope with the demands of a fast-paced, changing environment.

8.1 ESSENTIAL ADAPTOGENIC HERBS: ASHWAGANDHA AND HOLY BASIL

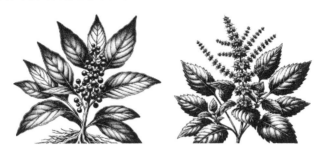

Ashwagandha and holy basil, revered adaptogens in Ayurvedic medicine, provide significant relief from the chronic stress and anxiety characteristic of today's fast-paced world. Ashwagandha, known scientifically as Withania somnifera or "Indian ginseng," reduces cortisol levels and mitigates the body's stress response, promoting mental clarity and emotional stability. Its active compounds, withanolides, help soothe and bolster resilience against psychological stressors, enhancing overall well-being. Similarly, holy basil, or Tulsi, known as "The Incomparable One," offers a range of health benefits from its aromatic leaves. It boosts the body's antioxidant defenses, reduces inflammation, and helps regulate blood sugar levels and metabolic disturbances caused by stress. Additionally, holy basil improves mental health by uplifting mood and fostering a sense of tranquility. Together, these herbs form a powerful duo for managing anxiety, supporting physical and psychological health, and promoting a balanced and peaceful existence in the face of modern challenges.

Practical Applications

To incorporate adaptogens like ashwagandha into daily routines, consider starting the day with a warm cup of milk (or a plant-based alternative) infused with a teaspoon of ashwagandha powder and sweetened with honey. A ritual like this in the morning—a moment of introspection before the day unfolds—sets a foundation of calm. Conversely, holy basil finds its best expression in a rejuvenating tea sipped in the evening as the sun's last rays kiss the horizon good-bye; steep the leaves in hot water, perhaps with a slice of ginger for warmth and a dash of lemon for zest. Tincture and capsule forms of these adaptogenic herbs are also available.

Moreover, the potential for adaptogens' pivotal role in mitigating stress is further enhanced when harmonized with lifestyle adjustments. Consider the act of journaling, a practice of reflection and mindfulness; when paired with the consumption of adaptogenic teas or tinctures, creating a ritual that marries introspection with the healing power of nature, you cultivate synergy and a deep-rooted and expansive resilience. Incorporating adaptogens into daily routines can significantly enhance one's quality of life by mitigating stress and promoting overall health and well-being.

Considerations and Interactions

When considering the use of ashwagandha and holy basil, two prominent adaptogenic herbs in Ayurvedic medicine, it is essential to understand their interactions and potential side effects to ensure safe and effective use. Ashwagandha, known for its ability to reduce cortisol and modulate stress responses, may interact with sedative medications or thyroid hormone pills, potentially enhancing their effects or altering thyroid hormone levels. Individuals with thyroid disorders or those taking sedatives should consult their healthcare provider before starting ashwagandha. Similarly, holy basil, which regulates blood sugar levels and has anti-inflammatory properties, could lower blood glucose too much when taken with diabetes medications. It may also enhance the effect of anticoagulant drugs, increasing the risk of bleeding. Both herbs can impact the liver's enzyme system in drug metabolism, which could alter the effectiveness of other medications. Pregnant or breastfeeding women should avoid using these herbs due to insufficient safety data. Therefore, individuals considering these herbs should discuss their use with a healthcare professional, particularly if they have pre-existing health conditions or are on medication, to tailor a regimen that acknowledges these interactions and respects the body's unique health needs.

For further reading, you can explore more details through the following links:

Ashwagandha: Everything You Need to Know

https://www.verywellhealth.com/ashwagandha-benefits-side-effects-and-more-7375260

Holy Basil Benefits: Ayurveda Herbal Medicine

https://www.verywellhealth.com/holy-basil-4766587

8.2 CHAMOMILE AND LAVENDER: HERBS FOR CRAFTING CALM, SOOTHING ANXIETY

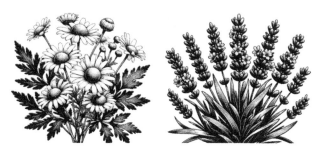

Chamomile and lavender, revered for their calming properties, serve as natural anxiolytics that significantly impact the nervous system and promote tranquility. Chamomile, primarily through the bioactive compound apigenin, binds to brain receptors like a key in a lock, initiating a neurological cascade that alleviates anxiety and encourages a return to calmness. This action provides not only temporary relief but a deep, enduring respite from anxiety, with regular consumption typically via tea, offering a gentle yet effective way to manage stress. Complementing chamomile, lavender's fragrance, rich in linalool and linalyl acetate, interacts with the brain's olfactory receptors to release calming neurotransmitters immediately, reducing stress and fostering a tranquil state of mind. Whether used in aromatherapy, diffused as an essential oil, or included in personal care products, lavender provides a direct, sensory path to peace, showcasing aromatics' powerful and holistic impact on emotional health. Chamomile and lavender form a robust duo that harnesses nature's potential to soothe the mind and promote psychological health and well-being in our fast-paced modern world.

Practical Applications

Chamomile and lavender are essential herbs in managing anxiety holistically, offering versatile applications in daily routines that cater to individual preferences and lifestyles. These herbs are most commonly consumed as teas, providing immediate soothing effects, but they are also available in tinctures and capsules for sustained relief throughout the day. For a more enhanced calming experience, blending chamomile and lavender with ginger and lemon balm can amplify the therapeutic benefits. Ginger adds warming properties that comfort the body, while lemon balm contributes a refreshing flavor that elevates the overall potency of the mixture. This herbal synergy soothes the nervous system to reduce anxiety and promotes a more relaxed state of mind, aiding in better navigation of daily stressors. Preparing this blend is a mindful activity, where measuring and steeping the herbs becomes a therapeutic ritual, infusing each sip of the beverage with intention and tranquility. Such rituals integrate these natural remedies into daily life, transforming drinking tea into a nurturing practice that supports a balanced and resilient approach to anxiety management.

Considerations and Interactions

While chamomile and lavender are known for their calming effects, you must consider their interactions with medications before incorporating them into an anxiety management routine. Both herbs, especially chamomile, may affect the efficacy of pharmaceuticals such as blood thinners, sedatives, and anti-anxiety medications. These interactions can occur because chamomile and lavender might potentiate or inhibit the effects of these drugs, leading to potentially unexpected outcomes. Therefore, consulting healthcare providers before using these herbs is crucial to ensure they complement existing treatments safely and effectively. Beyond their interactions, chamomile and lavender offer significant stress and anxiety relief benefits, suitable for long-term use due to their gentle, non-habit-forming properties. Regular consumption in forms like teas, tinctures, or capsules can help maintain a balanced mental state, gradually reducing the frequency and intensity of anxiety episodes. This proactive approach leverages the natural therapeutic properties of chamomile and lavender, fostering resilience and a sustained sense of calm in managing everyday stressors.

For further reading on chamomile, refer back to chapter 6; you can explore more details about lavender through the following link:

Lavender

https://www.drugs.com/mtm/lavender.html

8.3 HERBAL TEAS FOR RELAXATION AND SLEEP

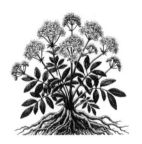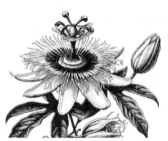

The ritual of brewing herbal teas for relaxation and sleep is a practice steeped in ancient tradition, serving as a pathway to wellness and serenity. This process is not just about the specific ingredients like valerian root and passionflower but also about the act of preparation and consumption, which becomes a calming, sensory experience. Valerian root, known for its earthy aroma, acts as a sedative by reducing the time it takes to fall asleep and enhancing sleep quality through its active compounds, valeric acid, and valerenol, which interact with brain receptors to quiet mental chatter. Passionflower complements this by easing anxiety and promoting deeper sleep through its effects on brain GABA (Gamma-aminobutyric acid) pathways. When combined in tea, these herbs synergistically create a potent elixir against insomnia and restlessness, honoring the body's natural need for rest.

Practical Application

To prepare the ideal herbal tea for sleep, attention to detail is crucial —from the quality of water and its temperature to the steeping time, each element plays a vital role in the alchemy of tranquility. Start with fresh, organic herbs to ensure potency and vitality. Boil water and allow it to cool slightly to avoid scorching the delicate herbal compounds, which can alter their flavor and effectiveness. Steep the valerian root and passionflower for seven to ten minutes to fully extract their sedative properties without introducing bitterness. Serve the tea in a pre-warmed cup, perhaps enhancing the flavor with a touch of honey or a slice of lemon. For a complete nighttime ritual, drink the tea in a tranquil environment, away from screens and daily distractions, in a space adorned with dim lights and soft textures, enhancing the calming effects. Such meticulous preparation and setting transform drinking tea into a holistic ritual that prepares the body and mind for restful sleep.

Considerations and Interactions

When integrating herbal teas such as valerian root and passionflower into a nighttime routine for relaxation and sleep, it's essential to consider potential interactions and individual sensitivities. Both valerian root and passionflower act as sedatives primarily through their influence on the central nervous system. Individuals currently using CNS depressants, such as benzodiazepines or certain types of antidepressants, should consult with healthcare providers before incorporating these teas, as the combined effect might excessively suppress the central nervous system. Additionally, while valerian root is generally safe, some people may experience side effects like headache, dizziness, or gastrointestinal disturbances. Though widely used for its calming effects, passionflower might not suit everyone; it is crucial to consider any existing medical conditions or medications that could interact negatively with these herbs. Pregnant or breastfeeding women, in particular, should avoid these herbs unless advised by a health professional, as their effects on fetal development or breast milk are not thoroughly studied. Ensuring the herbs' quality and freshness is also vital to prevent mold contamination or toxins that could negate their health benefits. By considering these factors, users can safely enjoy the therapeutic benefits of herbal teas while minimizing risks and enhancing their overall effectiveness in promoting restful sleep.

For further reading on valerian root and passionflower, you can explore more details through the following links:

Valerian: Uses For Sleep Aid, Side Effects and More
https://www.verywellhealth.com/what-you-need-to-know-about-valerian-88336

The Health Benefits of PassionFlower
https://www.verywellmind.com/how-is-passion-flower-used-to-treat-anxiety-3024970

8.4 CREATING YOUR STRESS-RELIEF HERBAL TOOLKIT

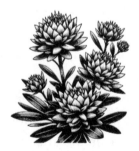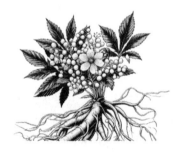

Crafting an effective herbal toolkit for stress relief requires a personalized approach, considering the specific types of stress you encounter. For acute stress situations, such as impending deadlines, an adaptogenic tea with rhodiola or ginseng can enhance mental performance and stress resistance. For more chronic stress resulting from ongoing emotional challenges, incorporating ashwagandha into your daily routine can help modulate your body's stress response and support adrenal health, making it ideal for sustained stress management. Augmenting these herbal remedies with mindfulness practices like focused breathing or meditation can enhance their effectiveness. Additionally, engaging in creative activities such as making chamomile and lavender bath bombs, blending massage oils with valerian root and ginger, or setting up a homemade aromatherapy diffuser with holy basil and lemon balm can provide a therapeutic and personalized touch to your stress relief regimen. This holistic approach helps alleviate stress symptoms and deepens your connection to personal health and well-being, making managing stress a more integrated and enjoyable part of life.

CHAPTER 9
FOCUSING THE LENS: ENHANCING MENTAL CLARITY

Leveraging nature's bounty, the judicious incorporation of specific herbs and fungi into our daily regimen can profoundly elevate our mental capabilities. Ginkgo Biloba, often celebrated as the Memory Herb, is instrumental in this blend, enhancing cerebral blood flow and neuronal activity, thereby bolstering memory and alertness. Complementing it, bacopa monnieri, known in traditional Ayurveda as Brahmi, is prized for its pronounced effects on memory retention and cognitive sharpness, aiding in effectively managing mental tasks. Rhodiola Rosea steps in as a fatigue fighter, enhancing mental stamina and resilience, which are crucial for maintaining concentration and productivity in high-stress scenarios. Similarly, lion's mane mushroom, a natural nootropic, plays a pivotal role by fostering the production of the *Nerve Growth Factor*, which is essential for maintaining and repairing neurons. Together, these natural substances form a potent cognitive-enhancing quartet that mitigates mental fatigue and promotes a sustainable, harmonious interaction with nature's healing rhythms, paving the way for enhanced mental clarity in our fast-paced, modern lives.

9.1 GINKGO BILOBA: THE MEMORY HERB

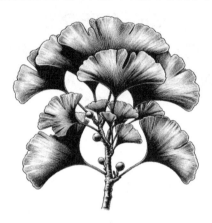

Ginkgo biloba, often revered as the Memory Herb, is a powerhouse of cognitive enhancement derived from one of the oldest tree species known to man—a "living fossil" that has thrived for over 270 million years. Its active compounds, flavonoids, and terpenoids, primarily drive its neuroprotective and cognitive benefits, mirroring its longevity. These compounds enhance cerebral blood flow, thereby improving the delivery of oxygen and nutrients essential for optimal brain function. This increased circulation helps sharpen memory and boost concentration by facilitating more efficient neural activities. Additionally, the antioxidant properties of ginkgo biloba robustly defend against oxidative stress, which contributes to age-related cognitive decline and neurodegenerative diseases. Through ongoing research, ginkgo continues to underscore its efficacy in improving physical health and cements its role in mental wellness by supporting and enhancing mental clarity and cognitive longevity.

Actions on Mental Clarity: Circulation

Ginkgo biloba, celebrated for its masterful enhancement of cerebral circulation, acts like a skilled conductor in the complex symphony of brain function. By improving the delivery of crucial nutrients and oxygen to the brain—much like a network of rivers efficiently distributing water—ginkgo ensures that every neuron is well-nourished and functional. The herb's flavonoids and terpenoids specifically widen blood vessels, boosting cerebral blood flow and enhancing cognitive abilities. This mechanism is pivotal as it guarantees brain cells receive the essential components to maintain mental sharpness and efficiency. An article published on *Mountsinai.org/* highlights that consistent use of ginkgo extract significantly improves blood flow in healthy adults, reinforcing its traditional use and potential as a therapeutic agent. This effect is crucial for reducing the risk of vascular-related cognitive impairments and bolstering strategies to enhance mental acuity and prevent cognitive decline, making ginkgo biloba a vital asset in cognitive health regimens and ongoing neurological research.

For further reading, you can explore more details through the following link:

Ginkgo Biloba
https://www.mountsinai.org/health-library/herb/ginkgo-biloba

Actions on Mental Clarity: Antioxidant Protection

Like the vast expanse of the night sky occasionally disturbed by storms, the mind, too, faces its disruptions in the form of oxidative stress—a damaging storm wrought by free radicals. Ginkgo biloba, known for its profound antioxidant properties, is a protective shield, guarding the neurons against the corrosive effects of these oxidative stresses. The potent flavonoids and terpenoid compounds found within ginkgo biloba play a critical role in this defense. These compounds effectively neutralize free radicals, thereby fortifying neural structures and ensuring the structural integrity of the mind remains intact. This protection is vital for maintaining cognitive functions and preventing the deterioration that can lead to disorders like dementia and Alzheimer's. Thus, ginkgo biloba supports mental performance and contributes to long-term brain health, making it an essential component of cognitive wellness regimens.

Actions on Mental Clarity: Memory and Concentration

Ginkgo Biloba, renowned for its precision in enhancing cognitive functions, acts akin to an expert tapestry weaver, meticulously integrating threads to form a complex and purposeful design. This herb significantly boosts mental clarity and focus by enhancing the intricate process of thought-weaving and memory retention. Its active components, particularly flavonoids and terpenoids, improve cerebral blood circulation, thus delivering more oxygen and essential nutrients to the brain cells. This surge in blood flow optimizes brain processes and supports cognitive functions across various age groups. Ginkgo Biloba has effectively enhanced cognitive performance, notably improving memory and concentration in young and older adults alike. This broad range of cognitive enhancement is valuable for countering age-related memory decline and boosting cognitive abilities in younger demographics. Additionally, ginkgo's antioxidant properties offer protection against oxidative stress, which contributes to cognitive deterioration by neutralizing harmful free radicals. By incorporating ginkgo biloba into daily health routines, individuals can foster improved cognitive understanding and resilience, preserving a sharp, active mind that enhances overall life quality as they age.

Practical Applications

Integrating ginkgo biloba into your daily regimen offers a versatile and effective way to enhance cognitive functions tailored to individual needs. Each method provides distinct advantages in various forms, such as capsules, teas, and tinctures. Capsules, for instance, offer a convenient and measured dose of ginkgo, making it easy to maintain consistency in intake. Teas provide a soothing and enjoyable way to consume ginkgo, potentially enhancing relaxation and mental clarity. Conversely, tinctures allow for rapid absorption and can be easily adjusted for dosage, catering to more immediate or specific cognitive demands. You can select the form of ginkgo that best addresses these issues by evaluating your current cognitive challenges, such as memory lapses, concentration difficulties, or mental fatigue. Personalizing your approach to ginkgo supplementation can lead to more targeted cognitive support, making it a mindful addition to your daily health practices.

Considerations and Interactions

Ginkgo Biloba, while highly beneficial for enhancing mental clarity and cognitive function, requires careful consideration due to its potent effects on blood circulation. Individuals taking anticoagulant medications or those with blood disorders should exercise caution, as ginkgo has properties that can intensify blood thinning. These individuals must consult healthcare professionals to tailor a safe dosage and monitor for potential interactions with other medications. The optimal use of ginkgo involves understanding its dual capacity to boost cerebral blood flow and provide antioxidative protection, enhancing memory, focus, and overall brain health. This alignment with the natural efficacy of ginkgo not only taps into the herb's ability to improve cognitive functions but also connects users with the enduring vitality mirrored in the longevity of the ginkgo tree itself. Thus, when used judiciously, ginkgo biloba is both a cognitive enhancer and a medium for experiencing nature's profound impact on health and well-being, illustrating a holistic approach to health that respects personal conditions and the broader natural context.

For further reading, you can explore more details by going back to chapter 3

9.2 BACOPA (BRAHMI): SHARPENING THE MIND

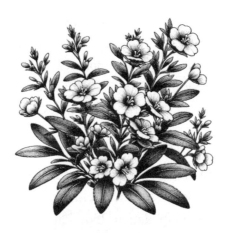

Bacopa monnieri, widely known and revered as Brahmi in the vast landscape of Ayurvedic medicine, stands as a beacon of cognitive enhancement. This esteemed herb has been integral to Ayurvedic practices for centuries. It is celebrated for remarkably improving memory, enhancing concentration, and providing a clarity of thought that scholars and spiritual seers have historically deemed essential. The texts and traditions of Ayurveda enshrine brahmi not just as a medicinal plant but as a vital tool for intellectual and spiritual empowerment.

The unique properties of brahmi make it a favorite among those seeking to boost cognitive functions due to its adaptogenic qualities that help mitigate stress, and its potential to enhance synaptic communication facilitates better learning and memory retention, qualities that are invaluable in the demanding pace of modern life. Furthermore, brahmi's continued relevance and popularity in contemporary wellness circles are a testament to its enduring efficacy and the deep cultural respect it commands. As research into its cognitive benefits expands, bacopa monnieri remains critical in pursuing mental excellence, echoing its historic use among ancient scholars and modern thinkers alike.

Actions on Mental Clarity: Neurotransmission

Bacopa monnieri's profound impact on neurotransmitter function is at the heart of its cognitive-enhancing effects. These effects involve the intricate modulation of the brain's chemical messengers, crucial in bridging synaptic gaps and enabling the rapid, seamless flow of information across the vast neural network. Bacopa's influence extends beyond mere amplification of these processes; it acts to refine and optimize the signaling pathways, much like fine-tuning a musical instrument to achieve perfect pitch.

The resulting enhancements manifest as a harmonious symphony of mental processes. Thoughts become more coherent and connect faster, akin to a well-rehearsed orchestra where each note contributes to a more prominent, precise melody. Memory recall improves, becoming sharper and more accessible, while the capacity for new learning is enhanced, allowing for quicker assimilation and retention of information. This sophisticated adjustment of neurotransmitter activity leads to more efficient cognitive functioning, fostering deeper insights and higher mental clarity. This precise tuning of the brain's communicative abilities is what makes bacopa monnieri a distinguished herb in the realm of cognitive enhancement.

Actions on Mental Clarity: Neuroprotection

Bacopa monnieri extends its benefits beyond enhancing neurotransmitter function. It is a formidable defense against the gradual onset of neurodegeneration—the progressive deterioration of neural pathways that can impact cognitive abilities over time. This herb acts as a protective bulwark, shielding the brain from the detrimental effects of oxidative stress and inflammation, which are vital contributors to the degenerative processes in neural tissues.

Oxidative stress occurs when an imbalance between free radicals and antioxidants in the body leads to cell damage. Bacopa contains powerful antioxidants that neutralize these free radicals, thereby reducing cellular damage and slowing the aging process of neurons. Additionally, its anti-inflammatory properties help mitigate the inflammatory responses in the brain, which can exacerbate neurodegenerative conditions. By calming these inflammatory pathways, bacopa helps preserve the structural and functional integrity of the brain's neural circuits.

This dual action of antioxidative and anti-inflammatory effects makes bacopa monnieri a cognitive enhancer and a vital agent in preventing age-related mental decline. It helps maintain long-term cognitive health, ensuring that the mind remains sharp and resilient against the natural wear and tear that comes with aging. This protective role of bacopa underscores its significance in neuroprotective strategies, providing a natural means to safeguard mental acuity and prolong cognitive vitality.

Adaptogenic Actions on Mental Clarity

Bacopa monnieri, known for its cognitive enhancement and neuro-protective effects, also excels as an adaptogen, effectively managing stress and boosting mental resilience. By stabilizing physiological processes and promoting homeostasis, particularly in stress responses, bacopa moderates cortisol secretion, which, when unchecked, can impair cognitive functions. This action preserves mental clarity, enabling better focus, memory retention, and problem-solving abilities under stress. Additionally, its adaptogenic properties mitigate immediate stressors and enhance long-term resilience against chronic stress, safeguarding mental health and preventing cognitive decline. Thus, bacopa is a vital tool for maintaining a clear and robust mind in the face of daily pressures.

Practical Applications

Bacopa monnieri is versatile in its application. It is available in various forms like tinctures, powders, and capsules, each offering unique advantages for incorporating into daily routines tailored to individual needs and lifestyles. Consider a morning ritual incorporating a bacopa supplement, its intake timed to precede the day's endeavors, laying a preemptive foundation of calm and focus. Or, if you're so culinary inclined, try incorporating bacopa powder into smoothies, infusing them with a touch of wellness. You can tailor each form of bacopa to fit different aspects of daily life, ensuring that you enjoy the cognitive benefits of this powerful herb in a manner that best suits your routine and dietary preferences. The optimal dosage should align with guidelines from experienced Ayurveda practitioners, who can provide personalized advice based on individual health profiles and needs.

Considerations and Interactions

Bacopa monnieri, deeply rooted in the wisdom of Ayurveda, serves as a cerebral sanctuary, enhancing mental clarity and easing the flow of thoughts, much like a river seamlessly reaching the sea. While we celebrate bacopa for its cognitive benefits, it is essential to acknowledge and respect the body's responses to herbal supplements. In some rare instances, bacopa may cause gastrointestinal discomfort, underscoring the importance of a personalized approach to its use. This potential side effect encourages users to be mindful of the dosage and the timing of consumption. Ideally, bacopa should be taken during the day, as its calming effects are most beneficial when aligned with daily activities and the body's natural rhythms that demand mental clarity. Such mindful integration helps maximize bacopa's cognitive benefits while minimizing discomfort, allowing the herb to truly enhance the mental acuity and focus needed to navigate the complexities of daily life.

For further reading, you can explore more details through the following link:

The Benefits of Bacopa

https://www.verywellhealth.com/the-benefits-of-bacopa-89039

9.3 RHODIOLA: COMBATING MENTAL FATIGUE

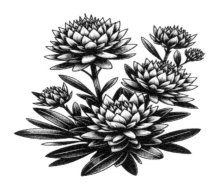

Rhodiola rosea is a formidable ally in the battle against mental fatigue, bridging the deep chasms of exhaustion that often plague modern life. This botanical marvel packs an intricate network of active compounds, including salidroside and rosavin, credited with its ability to rejuvenate a weary mind. Rhodiola offers much-needed solace for those constantly besieged by stress and the overwhelming demands of daily responsibilities. Its adaptogenic properties help enhance the body's resistance to stress, reducing fatigue and improving alertness and stamina. By bolstering the mind's resilience, rhodiola not only aids in combating immediate symptoms of mental exhaustion but also contributes to sustained cognitive vitality, making it an invaluable supplement for individuals looking to maintain high mental performance levels amidst the relentless pace of contemporary life.

Actions on Mental Clarity: Stress Resistance

Rhodiola rosea's exceptional capacity to bolster mental clarity and resistance to stress stems from its rich symphony of phytochemicals, which adeptly modulate the adrenal glands' response to stress triggers. These natural compounds, including salidroside and rosavin, regulate the release of cortisol, the body's primary stress hormone. When cortisol levels rise unchecked, they can cause significant physiological and psychological disarray, including disrupted sleep, impaired cognitive function, and increased anxiety. However, rhodiola's phytochemicals temper this response, maintaining cortisol at healthier levels and fostering a state of tranquility and sustained focus even in tumultuous situations. Research into rhodiola's stress-mitigating effects consistently shows a reduction in stress-induced fatigue, confirming its significant impact. This validation underscores the herb's powerful adaptogenic properties and highlights its role in enhancing cognitive function and mental resilience in daily stressors.

Actions on Mental Clarity: Fighting Fatigue

Rhodiola rosea emerges as a potent antidote to the pervasive tendrils of fatigue that can drain mental and physical vitality, dimming the brightness of consciousness. The herb works by enhancing oxygen utilization and boosting energy production at the cellular level, mechanisms critical for rekindling the body's dwindling embers of vitality. This increase in cellular energy translates into a more sustainable energy source that revitalizes the body and sharpens mental functions. As a result, individuals experiencing chronic fatigue find renewed energy and cognitive clarity, allowing them to navigate daily activities more efficiently and effectively. This dual action of rhodiola helps restore physical endurance and enhances mental alertness, making it a comprehensive solution for those seeking to reclaim their natural vitality and mental sharpness.

Actions on Mental Clarity: Enhancing Mood

Rhodiola rosea acts as a powerful catalyst in the delicate alchemy of mood regulation, interacting intricately with the body's chemical and electrical signals that govern emotional states. Specifically, rhodiola's influence targets the serotonergic and dopaminergic systems, critical architects of emotional equilibrium, joy, and satisfaction. Rhodiola carefully sculpts the mental landscape by modulating the activity within these neural pathways, much like a sculptor chipping away at the marble to reveal the statue within. This modulation helps to reshape the contours of mood disorders gently but effectively, unveiling a state of well-being that often lies obscured by the fluctuations of mental health challenges. This intervention results in a subtle yet profound elevation in mood, reflecting rhodiola's remarkable capacity for emotional stabilization. Individuals experiencing mood imbalances may find that rhodiola provides:

- *A natural, gentle uplift.*
- *Improvement in their overall well-being and emotional resilience.*
- *An invaluable herbal ally in the quest for mental harmony and psychological health.*

Practical Applications

Rhodiola rosea emerges as a dynamic and adaptable herb, ideal for integrating into daily routines through various forms tailored to individual needs and lifestyles. For those seeking a consistent and convenient way to harness rhodiola's benefits, capsules offer precise dosage, perfect for busy individuals aiming to maintain steady energy and mood throughout the day. Typically taken with meals, once or twice daily, capsules ensure a sustained release of the herb's active components. For immediate effects, tinctures offer rapid absorption and allow for flexible dosing that you can adjust based on daily stress levels and cognitive demands. A few drops in water or juice can swiftly enhance mental clarity and mood at critical times. Alternatively, rhodiola tea offers a more ritualistic and soothing experience, ideal for those preferring a gradual enhancement of cognitive and emotional well-being. Brewing the dried roots into tea can be a calming morning ritual or a revitalizing afternoon break, helping to fortify mental states and alleviate the day's stresses. Each method of rhodiola consumption leverages its adaptogenic properties to improve cognitive performance and emotional health, making it a valuable component of any wellness regimen.

Considerations and Interactions

Rhodiola rosea, a powerful adaptogen, is a refuge from stress and a source of mental vigor and emotional uplift. Experts recommend taking it in the morning or early afternoon to harness rhodiola's full potential without disrupting sleep. This timing capitalizes on its energizing effects during the hours most needed for mental engagement and physical activity. The herb's powerful influence on energy levels and mood makes timing crucial to avoid interference with nighttime rest. Although rhodiola is generally safe for most individuals, those with bipolar disorder or those using anticoagulants should exercise caution due to potential contraindications. It would be best if you personalized doses of rhodiola based on individual health profiles and the guidance of scientific evidence and healthcare professionals to ensure safety and efficacy. In doing so, rhodiola not only alleviates symptoms of stress and fatigue but also revitalizes the mind's resilience and restores emotional equilibrium, acting as a beacon of support in natural health supplements.

For further reading, you can explore more details through the following link:

The Health Benefits of Rhodiola
https://www.verywellmind.com/how-is-rhodiola-rosea-used-to-treat-anxiety-3024972

9.4 LION'S MANE MUSHROOM: NATURE'S BRAIN BOOSTER

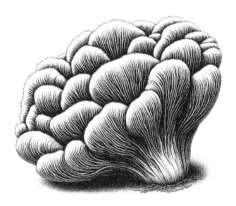

Lion's Mane Mushroom stands out in natural nootropics for its exceptional ability to support neural health and enhance mental clarity. This unique mushroom, characterized by its cascading, mane-like spines resembling a celestial lion, possesses remarkable cognitive-enhancing properties. In the world of herbal healing, the lion's mane actively stimulates the production of Nerve Growth Factor (NGF), making it highly valued. This protein plays a crucial role in neurons' growth, maintenance, and survival, positioning lion's mane as a critical agent in neural rejuvenation, promoting the repair and regeneration of nerve cells, which can lead to improved cognitive functions such as memory, focus, and overall mental clarity. Its tranquil appearance belies a potent force that not only boosts brain health but also opens new doors to enhanced neural function, making it a prized component in the arsenal of cognitive enhancers.

Actions on Mental Clarity: Brain Health

Lion's Mane Mushroom (Hericium erinaceus) plays a pivotal role in promoting brain health by actively stimulating the production of

Nerve Growth Factor (NGF). NGF is a vital protein essential for the survival, growth, and maintenance of neurons, acting as a critical component in the neural repair and regeneration processes. The bioactive compounds found within lion's mane, including hericenones and erinacines, are known to catalyze NGF synthesis, thereby directly influencing brain cell rejuvenation and combating the degenerative effects of aging and environmental stress on the brain. Scientific studies have specifically highlighted the mechanisms through which lion's mane exerts its effects, demonstrating that neural cells exposed to mushroom extracts show significantly enhanced NGF expression, underscoring the mushroom's potential in neuroprotective strategies but also its capability to improve cognitive functions and overall mental understanding, making it an invaluable resource in the field of neuro health and cognitive science.

For further reading, you can explore more details through the following link:

The Acute and Chronic Effects of Lion's Mane Mushroom Supplementation on Cognitive Function, Stress and mood in Young Adults: A Double-Blind, Parallel Groups, Pilot Study
https://www.ncbi.nlm.nih.gov/pmc/articles/PMC10675414/

Actions on Mental Clarity: Memory and Cognition

Lion's Mane Mushroom stimulates nerve growth and enhances memory and cognitive speed, earning it a widespread celebration. Research consistently validates these benefits, showing that lion's mane boosts day-to-day cognitive functions and protects against the onset of neurodegenerative diseases such as Alzheimer's and dementia. This dual capability makes the lion's mane a formidable guardian of neurological health. It enhances the brain's plasticity and the ability to adapt and reorganize itself, thereby improving memory retention and processing speed. These cognitive benefits are particularly significant as they suggest that regular consumption of lion's mane could offer long-term enhancements to brain function, fortifying it against the cognitive decline typically associated with aging. Thus, the lion's mane mushroom stands out in natural nootropics, offering immediate improvements in mental clarity and a strategic defense against future neurological challenges.

Actions on Mental Clarity: Mood and Anxiety

Lion's Mane Mushroom extends its cognitive benefits to include significant impacts on mood and anxiety, offering a natural respite for those grappling with mental unrest. Its adaptogenic properties are crucial in modulating the body's stress response. The lion's mane helps mitigate stress's physiological and psychological impacts by influencing hormonal balance and neural health. This modulation brings about a profound sense of calm, soothing the often-turbulent emotional states associated with anxiety. The result is a temporary alleviation of symptoms and a more sustained path to mental wellness. This calming effect enhances the mushroom's appeal as a holistic nootropic, capable of improving cognitive functions while fostering a tranquil mental environment, making it an invaluable aid for those seeking to maintain mental clarity and emotional stability in their daily lives.

Practical Applications

Lion's Mane's delicate, seafood-like flavor lends itself to many culinary preparations, from simple sautés to complex dishes, celebrating its texture and taste. Supplements may also offer a concentrated dose of the mushroom's bioactive compounds. Recommendations on daily intake and duration of use are flexible, guided by traditional practices and contemporary research, offering a framework for tailoring your mushroom use to your health narrative.

Lion's Mane takes a holistic approach to bolstering mental health, addressing both the physiological and the emotional, thus embodying the holistic philosophy that true wellness is not merely the absence of disease but the presence of harmony. The mushroom's contributions to brain health, mood stabilization, and neurological resilience offer hope for those seeking to elevate and balance their mental faculties and emotions—a testament to the boundless capacity for renewal inherent to the natural world.

Considerations and Interactions

While lion's mane mushroom offers many benefits for brain health, mood, and cognitive function, it is essential to consider potential interactions and individual responses when incorporating it into a wellness regimen. Generally well-tolerated, lion's mane may still interact with certain medications, particularly those affecting blood clotting and blood sugar levels, due to its potential antiplatelet and hypoglycemic effects. Individuals on medication for diabetes or blood thinners should consult with a healthcare provider before starting any supplement regimen that includes lion's mane. Additionally, as with any supplement, some people might experience mild digestive discomfort, especially when taken in large doses. Given its influence on NGF (Nerve Growth Factor)and hormonal balances, those with hormone-sensitive conditions should cautiously approach lion's mane. Tailoring the dosage and monitoring the body's response under professional guidance can help maximize the benefits of lion's mane while minimizing any adverse effects, ensuring this powerful natural nootropic's safe and effective use.

For further reading, you can explore more details through the following link:

Lion's Mane: Everything You Need to Know

https://www.verywellhealth.com/lions-mane-benefits-and-nutrition-profile-7498004

CHAPTER 10
THE WHISPER OF DREAMS HERBAL ALLIES FOR RESTFUL SLEEP

Many describe sleep as intricately weaving together our physical health and spiritual well-being. In herbal remedies, valerian and chamomile stand out as vigilant stewards of slumber, each playing a crucial role in this transformative process. Valerian is renowned for its potent sedative qualities, effectively calming the nervous system and alleviating the tension that often impedes sleep onset. This root's ability to transform restlessness into deep tranquility makes it a favored choice for those seeking a reliable pathway to restful nights. Chamomile complements valerian by providing a gentle, soothing effect, easing the mind from wakefulness into the comforting embrace of dreams. Its mild, calming properties are particularly suited for preparing the body and spirit for sleep, making these herbs a formidable duo in pursuing serene and refreshing slumber. Valerian and chamomile encapsulate the essence of nature's capacity to foster a peaceful transition from the day's liveliness to the rejuvenating silence of the night.

10.1 VALERIAN AND CHAMOMILE: NATURE'S SLEEP AIDS

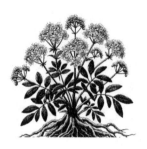 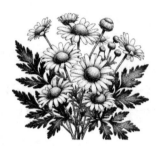

Valerian and chamomile are nature's quintessential sleep aids, revered throughout the ages for their remarkable abilities to foster deep and restorative sleep. Valerian's robust sedative qualities are particularly effective in quieting the restless mind and preparing the body for sleep. Its root, rich in compounds like valerenic acid, acts directly on the nervous system to reduce latency and encourage deeper sleep cycles. Chamomile complements valerian by offering a milder, soothing touch, with its warm, gentle embrace easing anxiety and promoting relaxation. As a duo, these herbs form a powerful alliance against the common adversaries of insomnia and nighttime restlessness, providing a natural, effective remedy that enhances sleep quality and prepares the body and mind for the rejuvenating power of a good night's rest.

Sleep-Promoting Actions: Sedative Properties

Valerian and chamomile are esteemed herbs that promote restful sleep by addressing mental and physical discomforts. Valerian acts on the central nervous system through its volatile oils and iridoids, such as valeric acid, sedating and calming the body to reduce the time it takes to fall asleep. On the other hand, chamomile contains:

- *Apigenin.*
- *An antioxidant that binds to brain receptors like a mild sedative.*
- *Easing the transition into sleep while alleviating anxiety and digestive discomfort.*

Together, these herbs offer a comprehensive approach to overcoming the hurdles interfering with a peaceful night's sleep, enhancing overall relaxation and well-being.

Sleep-Promoting Actions: Sleep Cycle Regulation

The sleep-wake cycle is a finely tuned dance of physiological rhythms, where any disruption can lead to significant sleep disturbances. Valerian and chamomile play crucial roles in preserving the harmony of this cycle. Valerian interacts with the brain's GABA receptors to enhance their inhibitory effects, facilitating the transition into sleep by calming neural activity. This interaction reduces the time to fall asleep and promotes a deeper, more restorative sleep. Chamomile complements this by also engaging with GABA(Gamma-aminobutyric acid) receptors. Still, it adds a layer of gentle sedation that smooths the transitions between the sleep stages—from the lightest phase to the deepest. This coordinated action of valerian and chamomile ensures that the sleep architecture remains intact and cyclical, allowing the body to progress through all necessary stages of sleep with dependable grace. The result is a sleep that genuinely rejuvenates and prepares the individual for the day ahead, underscoring the critical nature of these herbal allies in maintaining sleep health.

Sleep-promoting Actions: Anxiety Reduction

Anxiety frequently acts as a formidable barrier to sleep, setting the stage for restless nights and exhausted days. However, the herbal allies chamomile and valerian play pivotal roles in bridging the gap between persistent worry and restful slumber. Chamomile, with its gentle and soothing properties, provides relief from the grip of anxiety's anticipatory tendrils. It envelops the mind in a calming embrace, easing the mental tension and hyperarousal that often precede sleep. On the other hand, valerian targets the deeper undercurrents of anxiety with its potent sedative qualities. Its natural compounds act as a balm, soothing the agitated mind and dampening the overactive nervous responses associated with anxiety. Together, chamomile and valerian mediate a truce between relentless thoughts and the need for rest and create a conducive environment for sleep, allowing the body and mind to heal and recover through the night.

Practical Applications

Integrating valerian and chamomile into your nightly routine can significantly enhance your sleep quality, each herb offering distinct benefits suited to different sensitivities and preferences. When using valerian, it's advisable to begin with a modest dose to observe its specific effects on your individual body and sleep rhythms. A practical approach is to brew tea from its roots, consuming it about an hour before bedtime. Doing this allows you to monitor and adjust the dosage according to your response, ensuring an optimal balance between efficacy and comfort. Chamomile, on the other hand, is more forgiving and versatile. You can enjoy multiple cups of chamomile tea throughout the evening, as its gentle sedative properties tend to deepen with each serving, gradually easing you into a state of relaxed readiness for sleep, making chamomile an ideal herb for those seeking a milder, more gradually intensifying approach to sleep induction. These herbs can be critical components of a calming pre-sleep ritual, setting the stage for a restful night.

Considerations and Interactions

While valerian and chamomile are renowned for their sleep-promoting properties, it is essential to consider their interactions and potential side effects, primarily when used with other medications. Valerian, known for its potent sedative effects, can interact with benzodiazepines, sedatives, and other medications that depress the central nervous system, potentially exacerbating their impact and leading to excessive drowsiness or impaired motor functions. Therefore, those taking CNS (central nervous system) depressants should consult a healthcare provider before incorporating valerian into their regimen. Similarly, chamomile, while milder, can interfere with anticoagulant medications due to its blood-thinning properties, posing a risk of bleeding, particularly in individuals on warfarin or other blood thinners. Additionally, both herbs may cause allergic reactions in susceptible individuals, especially those with allergies to plants in the Asteraceae family, which includes chamomile. Given these considerations, it is crucial to approach these herbal remedies cautiously, ideally under the guidance of a healthcare professional who can advise on appropriate dosages and potential interactions with other medications or health conditions, ensuring the safe and effective use of these natural sleep aids.

We looked at chamomile earlier in chapter 7; for further reading on valerian, refer to chapter 8

10.2 LAVENDER: THE SCENT OF RELAXATION

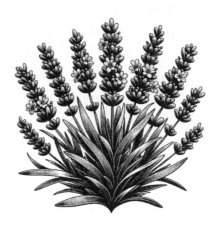

Lavender is a botanical sovereign revered for its profound ability to instill tranquility. Its potent aroma, characterized by a symphony of soothing compounds such as linalool and linalyl acetate, is pivotal in calming the nervous system. This gentle yet effective interaction quiets the constant noise of daily life, creating a peaceful environment that allows for a state of serene alertness. The unique aromatic profile of lavender reduces anxiety and stress and enhances cognitive functions, making it an ideal companion for those seeking a mental reset amid a hectic schedule. As it diffuses through the air, lavender's fragrance works to soothe the mind and foster a sense of well-being, proving itself a powerful ally in pursuing mental clarity and relaxed focus.

Sleep-Promoting Actions: Aromatherapy

The science and discipline of aromatherapy is as ancient as it is modern—and lavender is a cornerstone of its practice. Rigorous studies have illuminated the pathways through which lavender's scent modulates the body's response to stress: inhaling the herb's fragrance activates the oldest part of the brain, the limbic system, where emotions and memories reside; this signals the release of neurotransmitters, chemical messengers that traverse the neural landscape, carrying messages of relaxation to every corner of the body. Researchers have observed a significant decrease in cortisol levels—the precursor of stress— in those who partake of the herb's aroma.

Sleep-Promoting Actions: Sleep Duration

Lavender's characteristic aroma extends its benefits beyond merely easing stress—it also significantly enhances sleep duration, particularly the length of deep sleep, which is crucial for physical and mental restoration. The soothing scent of lavender acts as a natural lullaby, quieting the restless mind and promoting prolonged periods of deep sleep. This sleep phase is essential for the body's healing and cognitive restoration, making lavender an invaluable sleep aid. Clinical trials have consistently supported these effects, demonstrating that environments infused with lavender deepen sleep and increase overall restfulness. Such studies reveal a clear, direct correlation between the calming aroma of lavender and improved sleep quality, showcasing lavender's potent therapeutic properties in fostering a night of sleep that revitalizes and rejuvenates the body and mind.

For further reading, you can explore more details through the following link:

Effect of Inhaled Lavender and Sleep Hygiene on Self-Reported Issues: A Randomized Control Trial

https://www.ncbi.nlm.nih.gov/pmc/articles/PMC4505755/

Practical Applications

Lavender's versatility in application allows it to cater to individual preferences and needs, making it a multifaceted aid for relaxation and sleep. Oil diffusers, for instance, vaporize lavender essence, filling living spaces with a soothing aroma that converts any room into a sanctuary of peace. For those who prefer a more personal approach, pillow sprays infused with lavender provide a direct, intimate experience, with each inhalation at bedtime deepening relaxation. Topically, lavender can be applied through body lotions, where the oils absorb into the skin, utilizing the body's largest organ to diffuse its calming effects. Beyond these methods, lavender can also be enjoyed as a soothing tea, offering a warm, comforting ritual before sleep, or used in more concentrated forms like capsules or tinctures for those seeking precise dosages. Each application method uniquely contributes to deep relaxation, paving the way for a night of profound, restorative sleep.

Considerations and Interactions

While lavender is renowned for its calming properties, it is essential to approach its use with mindfulness, mainly due to the potent nature of lavender oil. For those considering topical applications, it's crucial to recognize that lavender oil can cause reactions in individuals with sensitive skin, although generally benign. Conducting a patch test before wider use can help determine compatibility, ensuring the journey to relaxation remains smooth and free from irritants. Additionally, the concentrated essence of lavender oil, whether inhaled, sprayed, or applied directly to the skin, often requires dilution to mitigate its intensity and maximize its benefits safely. This careful handling is not only a precaution but also a form of respect for the powerful effects of this benevolent herb, underscoring the need to honor the potency nature provides in even its most soothing forms.

You can review details on lavender through the link in chapter 8:

10.3 LEMON BALM: EASING THE MIND FOR BETTER SLEEP

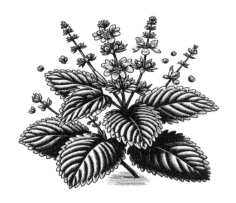

With its lush green leaves and subtle lemon fragrance, lemon balm emerges as a gentle yet powerful herbal remedy for calming the mind and enhancing sleep quality. This herb is remarkably esteemed for its natural ability to smooth the ripples of stress and anxiety, effectively clearing the way to the sanctuary of restful sleep. Its soothing properties make lemon balm a valued ally in the battle against restlessness and insomnia, offering a natural solution for those seeking a peaceful escape from the day's worries. Whether used in teas, as an essential oil, or in other therapeutic forms, lemon balm's delightful aroma and calming effects can transform your bedtime routine into a tranquil journey toward deep, restorative slumber.

Sleep-Promoting Actions: Stress and Anxiety Relief

Lemon Balm, scientifically known as Melissa officinalis, stands out for its potent compounds, such as rosmarinic acid and a rich bouquet of terpenes, which expertly engage and modulate the nervous system. These compounds work with the precision of a skilled maestro, subtly adjusting mood and significantly alleviating the stress and anxieties that keep the mind alert and awake. This herb's soothing effects create a calming internal environment where the day's chaos gently fades into the background, replaced by a tranquil serenity that ushers in the onset of sleep. As it eases the mind and soothes the spirit, lemon balm sets the stage for a night of deep, restorative sleep, making it an invaluable herb for those who struggle with sleeplessness due to mental burdens and restlessness.

Practical Applications

To harness the sleep-promoting benefits of lemon balm, consider starting with a soothing tea or a potent tincture, each offering a unique approach to relaxation and sleep preparation. Select high-quality, fresh, or dried lemon balm leaves for the tea—vital for maximizing the remedy's efficacy. Measure a spoonful of leaves for each cup of boiling water, steeping the mixture for five to ten minutes, releasing the leaves' full spectrum of flavors and calming properties, transforming the hot water into a warm, drowsy embrace. If you desire a more concentrated effect, consider using lemon balm tinctures as a powerful alternative. A few drops under the tongue can quickly deliver the herb's calming properties directly into the bloodstream. Whether you choose tea or tincture, preparing lemon balm becomes a meditative ritual, focusing the mind on relaxation and sleep. Each step in the preparation is an act of deliberate self-care, setting the stage for a restful night.

Considerations and Interactions

Lemon Balm earns wide recognition for its safety and efficacy in soothing anxiety and stress and promoting better sleep. However, like any herb, you should use it judiciously to avoid any potential side effects, which, though rare, usually manifest as mild digestive discomfort. These considerations highlight the importance of consulting with healthcare professionals, especially for those who may be taking other medications, to ensure that lemon balm serves as an aid to sleep rather than a complication. Mindful dosing, tailored to the body's response, is crucial in leveraging lemon balm's benefits without overstepping its bounds. Furthermore, lemon balm's ability to work synergistically with other complementary botanicals enhances its role as a cornerstone of natural sleep support. The ritual of preparing lemon balm, whether as tea or tincture, integrates intention with action, creating a holistic journey toward sleep that encompasses the cessation of wakefulness and the cultivation of deep, peaceful tranquility.

For further reading, you can explore more details through the following link:

Everything You Need to Know About Lemon Balm

https://www.verywellhealth.com/the-health-benefits-of-lemon-balm-89388

10.4 PASSIONFLOWER: AN HERBAL ROUTE TO RESTFUL NIGHTS

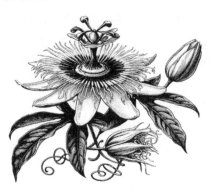

With its captivating blooms and intricate tendrils, passionflower is more than just a visual delight; it is a potent herbal remedy for insomnia and restlessness. This striking plant goes beyond its ornamental value to be a powerful key to unlocking deep and restful sleep. Its efficacy in calming the mind and easing the body into a state of relaxation allows it to breach the threshold of dreams effectively. Passionflower works by increasing levels of gamma-aminobutyric acid (GABA) in the brain, which lowers brain activity and helps to alleviate anxiety, ultimately fostering a tranquil environment conducive to sleep, making passionflower an invaluable herbal route for those seeking to escape the grip of sleepless nights and embrace the restorative power of peaceful slumber.

Sleep-Promoting Actions: Settling the Mind

Passionflower (Passiflora incarnata) promotes restful sleep by enhancing the GABA (gamma-aminobutyric acid) neurotransmitter system, essential for calming the brain. It increases GABA levels in the brain, reducing neuronal activity and helping to quiet the mind. The bioactive compounds in passionflower improve GABA binding to its receptors, soothing anxiety and easing the body into deep sleep. Supported by research confirming its role in boosting GABAergic activity, passionflower effectively manages insomnia. It ensures a restful and rejuvenating night's sleep, making it a valuable component of any herbal sleep-aid toolkit.

Sleep-Promoting Actions: Fighting Insomnia

Passionflower has proven to be a formidable adversary against insomnia and other sleep disorders, offering significant relief for those caught in the grip of sleepless nights. Individuals who have insomnia have reported notable improvements in sleep quality after using passionflower. The benefits of passionflower extend beyond simply increasing the duration of sleep; it also hastens the onset of sleep and deepens the experience, enhancing the quality of rest. This herb's impact makes each moment spent asleep more effective for rejuvenation, transforming restless nights into periods of profound, restorative slumber. By targeting the underlying mechanisms of sleep at both quantitative and qualitative levels, passionflower ensures that sleep becomes a genuinely healing experience, reinforcing its role as a critical natural remedy in managing sleep disturbances.

Practical Applications

Incorporating passionflower into your nightly routine can significantly enhance your journey toward restful sleep. One effective method is brewing a comforting tea from the passionflower's dried flowers and leaves, allowing the beverage's warmth to serve as a gentle prelude to sleep. Alternatively, passionflower tinctures provide a convenient option for those seeking a more direct and potent approach. These concentrated extracts offer a quicker route to relaxation, making them particularly beneficial for individuals experiencing difficulty in unwinding before bedtime. Passionflower should ideally be consumed during the hours leading up to sleep, aligning its peak effects with the body's natural rhythm of winding down for the night. Integrating passionflower into your evening routine helps create a soothing ritual that promotes relaxation and supports a peaceful transition into rejuvenating sleep, filling each night with tranquility and restorative rest.

Considerations and Interactions

Considering the potency and efficacy of passionflower in promoting restful sleep, it's essential to approach its integration with other herbs and medications with care. While passionflower is generally well-tolerated and has few known interactions, it's advisable to consult a healthcare professional before combining it with other calming herbs or supplements, especially if you're already taking medications or have underlying health conditions. Although passionflower is considered safe for most individuals, potential interactions may exist, particularly when combined with medications that affect the central nervous system or have sedative effects. Additionally, you should exercise caution when combining passionflower with other substances that induce drowsiness, as this may enhance the sedative effects and lead to excessive drowsiness or dizziness. By seeking guidance from a healthcare provider, you can ensure that passionflower is integrated safely and effectively into your sleep regimen, maximizing its benefits and minimizing potential risks or interactions, as discussed earlier.

For further reading, you can explore more details through the following link:

The Health Benefits of Passion Flower
https://www.verywellmind.com/how-is-passion-flower-used-to-treat-anxiety-3024970

CONCLUSION

As we reflect on our exploration of herbal medicine, it becomes evident how deeply intertwined these ancient practices are with modern approaches to health and wellness. The journey has not only highlighted the vast array of herbs, each with unique properties and benefits, but also their significant role in historical and cultural contexts. Delving into various herb categories has revealed a transformative potential when applied to contemporary health issues. This exploration has underscored the seamless integration of the ancient wisdom of herbal medicine into our daily lives, showcasing its relevance and vitality in offering health benefits and fostering a deeper connection to nature's natural rhythms and gifts.

This renewed understanding invites us to forge a deeper and more nurturing relationship with the natural world. Through learning about individual herbs and their specific roles in enhancing health and wellness, we have seen how these natural allies can guide us toward improved health and a more harmonious balance with our environment. The holistic approach advocated by herbal medicine provides remedies and promotes a way of living that encompasses physical, mental, and environmental health and well-being. By embracing these practices, we access age-old knowledge that remains as pertinent today as it was centuries ago, promising transformative benefits and a sustainable path forward in our health journeys.

Throughout this book, we have built a solid foundation for engaging with herbal healing, traversing specific herbs' rich cultural and practical landscapes. Each herb has been selected because it supports targeted areas of our health and well-being—whether boosting immunity, reducing stress, improving digestion, or enhancing sleep quality. The insights gained into the diverse applications of these herbs deepen our understanding of each herb's unique properties and highlight the interconnectedness of our body's systems with the natural world. This comprehensive exploration informs and empowers us to effectively incorporate these natural solutions into our lives.

Further, we've delved into practical applications of herbs, emphasizing their versatility in enhancing health and wellness in our daily living. This practical guidance equips us with the knowledge to seamlessly integrate herbal practices into everyday routines, fostering a holistic approach to health and wellness. Whether incorporating herbal supplements, or preparing therapeutic teas, the strategies discussed pave the way for harnessing the full potential of herbal medicine, contributing to a lifestyle that prioritizes sustainable health and a deep connection to earth's healing powers.

One of the core themes of this journey is the empowerment that comes from taking an active role in one's health and wellness. Armed with comprehensive knowledge and practical tools, you are well-prepared to embark on a path that aligns with your needs and lifestyle. This journey encourages experimentation and attunement to your body's responses, allowing you to customize herbal solutions that enhance your well-being. The empowerment stems from the understanding that using natural resources like herbs can significantly influence positive health outcomes.

As you close this book, view it not as an end but as the beginning of a broader exploration into herbal wellness. Continue to seek knowledge and connect with communities that share your interest in herbal medicine. There are countless resources, workshops, and enthusiastic fellow herbalists eager to share their insights and experiences, which can further enrich your understanding and application of herbal practices. Engage actively with these opportunities, remaining open and curious. The world of herbal wisdom is vast and continually evolving, offering endless possibilities for learning and growth.

In closing, let this book be a source of inspiration and a tool for empowerment as you continue to explore the profound benefits of herbal medicine. Embrace this ongoing journey with enthusiasm and a spirit of discovery, letting the plants around you guide you toward a healthier, more harmonized life. Thank you for allowing me to be a part of your health and wellness journey, and may you find deep fulfillment and empowerment in these practices as you forge a path toward living in greater harmony with the natural world.

Warmly and with heartfelt thanks,

Rami Archer

SHARING THE KNOWLEDGE YOU'VE LEARNED

Now you have everything you need to unlock wellness with natural herbal remedies,for better health, it's time to pass on your newfound knowledge and show other readers where they can find the same help.

Imagine how amazing it feels to share something special with others, especially when it can make a big difference in their lives. That's what we're inviting you to do.

Your experience with *"Unlocking Wellness: Natural Herbal Remedies for Diseases" by Rami Archer* is valuable . Sharing your thoughts can help others discover the same benefits you've found.

Leaving a review takes just a minute. Would you help someone you've never met by leaving a review?

Your review can guide others who are curious about natural health, just like you were. Here's why your review matters:

- *It helps one more person find natural ways to stay healthy.*
- *It supports one more family in using herbal remedies.*
- *It boosts confidence for one more person in their health choices.*
- *It inspires one more reader to learn something new.*
- *It makes one more dream of good health come true.*

To share your thoughts, all you have to do is leave a review. It costs nothing and takes less than a minute, but it can change someone's life.

Simply scan the QR code below to leave your review:

https://www.amazon.com/review/review-your-purchases/?asin= B0DCGLTXJL

If you love helping others, you're our kind of person. Welcome to the club. You're one of us.

Thank you from the bottom of my heart for being part of this journey. Your review can keep the game alive for so many others.

Your biggest fan, Rami Archer

PS. *Remember, when you share something of value with others, you become even more valuable to them. If you believe this book can help someone you know, don't hesitate to pass it on!*

REFERENCE

1 Lillehei, A. S., Halcón, L. L., Savik, K., & Reis, R. (2015). Effect of inhaled lavender and Sleep Hygiene on Self-Reported Sleep Issues: a randomized controlled trial. *the Journal of Alternative and Complementary Medicine/Journal of Alternative and Complementary Medicine, 21*(7), 430–438. https://doi.org/10.1089/acm.2014.0327

2 Rdn, B. L. M. (2023, April 27). *What are the benefits of milk thistle?* Verywell Health. https://www.verywellhealth.com/the-benefits-of-milk-thistle-88325

3 Rdn, H. C. M. (2023, November 8). *Cat's claw: a traditional herbal remedy that should be used with caution.* Verywell Health. https://www.verywellhealth.com/cats-claw-benefits-and-safety-8379773

4 *Rdn, B. L. M. (2023b, May 16). Everything you need to know about Coriander. Verywell Health. https://www.verywellhealth.com/coriander-7488672*

5 *Rdn, B. L. M. (2023d, June 5). Echinacea: everything you need to know. Verywell Health. https://www.verywellhealth.com/echinacea-benefits-side-effects-and-more-7503379*

6 *Rdn, B. L. M. (2023c, May 23). Fennel and fennel seeds: A look at the benefits. Verywell Health. https://www.verywellhealth.com/fennel-and-fennel-seeds-benefits-uses-and-more-7495392*

7 *Pugle, M. (2023, June 14). Kratom: Weighing the benefits and risks. Verywell Health. https://www.verywellhealth.com/kratom-7499659*

8 *Rdn, R. C. W. M. (2024, April 5). Turmeric and its antioxidant curcumin. Verywell Health. https://www.verywellhealth.com/turmeric-curcumin-benefits-7110668*

9 *Bcps, R. P. P. B. B. (2023, June 21). Health uses of ginger. Verywell Health. https://www.verywellhealth.com/ginger-health-uses-nutrition-and-more-7487136#:~*

10 *Nutrients (2023, 15(22), 4842; https://doi.org/10.3390/nu15224842*

11 *Rdn, B. L. M. (2024, May 31). Boswellia: a supplement to relieve inflammation? Verywell Health. https://www.verywellhealth.com/the-health-benefits-of-boswellia-89549#:~*

12 *Bcps, R. P. P. B. B. (2023b, November 7). Bitter Melon: Benefits and Nutrition. Verywell Health. https://www.verywellhealth.com/bitter-melon-benefits-and-nutrition-7505756#:~*

13 *Rd, B. C. (2023, June 29). Evidenced-Based health benefits of cinnamon. Verywell Health. https://www.verywellhealth.com/cinnamon-7505730*

14 Rdn, R. C. W. M. (2023, June 11). Hawthorn: Benefits and Nutrition. Verywell Health. https://www.verywellhealth.com/the-benefits-of-hawthorn-89057

15 PharmD, M. N. (2022, December 21). What is Allicin? Verywell Health. https://www.verywellhealth.com/the-benefits-of-allicin-88606

16 Bcps, R. P. P. B. B. (2023a, April 25). Potential health benefits of eleuthero. Verywell Health. https://www.verywellhealth.com/health-benefits-of-eleuthero-89449

17 Rdn, B. L. M. (2024a, March 31). What are the health benefits of Cordyceps supplements? Verywell Health. https://www.verywellhealth.com/benefits-of-cordyceps-89441

18 Poppy Uses, Benefits & Dosage Herbal Database. (n.d.). Drugs.com. https://www.drugs.com/npp/poppy.html#24362742

19 Clark, A., PhD. (2023, July 29). 11 Dandelion root benefits. Verywell Health. https://www.verywellhealth.com/the-benefits-of-dandelion-root-89103

20 PharmD, T. T. (2023, April 28). Kava: Everything you need to know. Verywell Health. https://www.verywellhealth.com/kava-uses-risks-and-more-7481255

21 Rdn, B. L. M. (2023c, June 28). What to know about the benefits of peppermint leaf. Verywell Health. https://www.verywellhealth.com/peppermint-uses-dosage-and-more-7511339

22 Ld, L. a. M. R. (2024, March 20). What is Astragalus good for? Verywell Health. https://www.verywellhealth.com/astragalus-what-should-i-know-about-it-89410

23 Rdn, B. L. M. (2023a, April 19). Ashwagandha: Everything you need to know. Verywell Health. https://www.verywellhealth.com/ashwagandha-benefits-side-effects-and-more-7375260

24 Bcps, R. P. P. B. B. (2023c, July 5). Holy Basil Benefits: Ayurveda Herbal Medicine. Verywell Health. https://www.verywellhealth.com/holy-basil-4766587

25 Rdn, B. L. M. (2023b, February 11). Valerian: Uses as sleep aid, side effects, and more. Verywell Health. https://www.verywellhealth.com/what-you-need-to-know-about-valerian-88336

26 Clark, A., PhD. (2023a, May 30). Everything you need to know about Lemon balm. Verywell Health. https://www.verywellhealth.com/the-health-benefits-of-lemon-balm-89388

27 JAMAICAN DOGWOOD: Overview, uses, side effects, precautions, interactions, dosing and reviews. (n.d.). https://www.webmd.com/vitamins/ai/ingredientmono-529/jamaican-dogwood

28 Andrographis Uses, Benefits & Dosage Herbal Database. (n.d.). Drugs.com. https://www.drugs.com/npp/andrographis.html

29 Fand, J. L. M. R. C. (2023, September 28). What is Elderberry good for? Verywell Health. https://www.verywellhealth.com/elderberry-for-colds-and-flu-can-it-help-89559

30 *Willow Bark Uses, Benefits & Side Effects Herbal Database.* (n.d.). Drugs.com. https://www.drugs.com/npc/willow-bark.html

31 Wong, C. (2022, August 17). *The health benefits and side effects of ginkgo biloba.* Verywell Mind. https://www.verywellmind.com/ginkgo-what-should-you-know-about-it-88329

32 Rdn, B. L. M. (2023a, February 11). *Valerian: Uses as sleep aid, side effects, and more.* Verywell Health. https://www.verywellhealth.com/what-you-need-to-know-about-valerian-88336

33 *PharmD, M. N. (2023b, June 29). Lion's Mane: Everything You Need to Know. Verywell Health. https://www.verywellhealth.com/lions-mane-benefits-and-nutrition-profile-7498004*

34 *Cuncic, A., MA. (2022b, December 1). The health benefits of Rhodiola. Verywell Mind. https://www.verywellmind.com/how-is-rhodiola-rosea-used-to-treat-anxiety-3024972*

35 Bcps, R. P. P. B. B. (2023a, April 13). *Top benefits of Bacopa.* Verywell Health. https://www.verywellhealth.com/the-benefits-of-bacopa-89039

36 Parker, J. (n.d.). Echinacea and the immune system. *Echinacea and the Immune System.* https://www.nottingham.ac.uk/biosciences/documents/burn/2006/echinacea-and-the-immune-system--juliet-parker.pdf

37 *Cuncic, A., MA. (2022, September 13). The health benefits of Passion flower. Verywell Mind. https://www.verywellmind.com/how-is-passion-flower-used-to-treat-anxiety-3024970*

38 *Lavender Uses, Side Effects & Warnings. (n.d.). Drugs.com. https://www.drugs.com/mtm/lavender.html*

39 Immune-Boosting Foods For Cold And Flu Season – Long Island Weekly. https://longislandweekly.com/immune-boosting-foods-for-cold-and-flu-season/

40 PharmD, M. N. (2023, June 1). *German Chamomile: Uses, Safety, & More.* Verywell Health. https://www.verywellhealth.com/the-benefits-of-chamomile-89436

41 *Gentian Uses, Benefits & Dosage Herbal Database.* (n.d.). Drugs.com. https://www.drugs.com/npp/gentian.html

42 Holy Basil/Tulsi (Ocimum Tenuiflorum/Ocimum Sanctum Linn) – Greal. https://www.greal.co/pages/holy-basil-tulsi-ocimum-tenuiflorum-ocimum-sanctum-linn

43 *Jaclyn Goodrich | U-M LSA International Institute.* (n.d.). https://ii.umich.edu/ii/people/all/g/gaydojac.html

44 Lee, H., & Park, W. (2010). Public Health Policy for Management of Hepatitis B virus infection: Historical review of recommendations for Immunization. *Public Health Nursing, 27*(2), 148–157. https://doi.org/10.1111/j.1525-1446.2010.00842.x

45 Sah, A., Naseef, P. P., Kuruniyan, M. S., Jain, G., Zakir, F., & Aggarwal, G. (2022). A comprehensive study of therapeutic applications of chamomile. *Pharmaceuticals, 15*(10), 1284. https://doi.org/10.3390/ph15101284

46 Vanaspatiteam. (2023, April 17). *Herbal Spotlight: Passionflower.* Vana Tisanes. https://vanatisanes.com/2018/10/30/passionflower/

47 Mirzaee, F., Hosseini, A., Jouybari, H. B., Davoodi, A., & Azadbakht, M. (2017). Medicinal, biological and phytochemical properties of Gentiana species. *Journal of Traditional and Complementary Medicine, 7*(4), 400–408. https://doi.org/10.1016/j.jtcme.2016.12.013

48 What is gastroesophageal reflux? | Advanced Surgical & Bariatrics of NJ. Advanced Surgical & Bariatrics of NJ. (2024, January 18). *What is gastroesophageal reflux? | Advanced Surgical & Bariatrics of NJ.* https://www.bariatricsurgerynewjersey.com/patient-resources/frequently-asked-questions/what-is-gastroesophageal-reflux/

49 Ajdigi. (2023, January 3). *Ratchet plant benefits.* Live to Plant. https://livetoplant.com/ratchet-plant-benefits/

50 Lad, N. (2023). The gut microbiota as a novel nutritional target to influence systemic inflammation associated with prevalent health disorders. https://core.ac.uk/download/580089943.pdf

51 Rezzani, R., & Franco, C. (2019). Curcumin as a Therapeutic Strategy in Liver Diseases. Nutrients, 11(10), 2498

52 Das, G., Shin, H., & Patra, J. (2022). Key Health Benefits of Korean Ueong Dry Root Extract Combined Silver Nanoparticles. International Journal of Nanomedicine, 17(), 4261-4275.

53 Strand, J. (2022). Distinctive Detoxification: The Case for Including the Microbiome in Detox Strategy. Integrative Medicine, 21(4), 26-30.

54 Bonaterra, G. A., Heinrich, E., Kelber, O., Weiser, D., Metz, J., & Kinscherf, R. (2010). Anti-inflammatory effects of the willow bark extract STW 33-I (Proaktiv®) in LPS-activated human monocytes and differentiated macrophages. *Phytomedicine, 17*(14), 1106–1113. https://doi.org/10.1016/j.phymed.2010.03.022

55 Federico, A., Dallio, M., & Loguercio, C. (2017). Silymarin/Silybin and chronic liver disease: a marriage of many years. *Molecules/Molecules Online/Molecules Annual, 22*(2), 191. https://doi.org/10.3390/molecules22020191

56 *Journal of Clinical Gastroenterology* 48(6):p 505-512, July 2014. | *DOI:* 10.1097/MCG.0b013e3182a88357

57 *Dandelion root Benefits, uses, interactions and side effects - Dr. Axe.* (2023, August 15). Dr. Axe. https://draxe.com/nutrition/dandelion-root/

58 Farzaei, M. H., Zobeiri, M., Parvizi, F., El-Senduny, F. F., Marmouzi, I., Coy-Barrera, E., Naseri, R., Nabavi, S. M., Rahimi, R., & Abdollahi, M. (2018). Curcumin in liver Diseases: A systematic review of the cellular mechanisms of oxidative stress and clinical perspective. *Nutrients, 10*(7), 855. https://doi.org/10.3390/nu10070855

59 Shara, M., & Stohs, S. J. (2015d). Efficacy and Safety of White Willow Bark (Salix

alba) Extracts. *PTR. Phytotherapy Research/Phytotherapy Research*, 29(8), 1112–1116. https://doi.org/10.1002/ptr.5377

60 Bonaterra, G. A., Kelber, O., Weiser, D., Metz, J., & Kinscherf, R. (2011). In vitro anti-proliferative effects of the willow bark extract STW 33-I. *Arzneimittel-Forschung*, 60(06), 330–335. https://doi.org/10.1055/s-0031-1296296

61 Free Research Project. (2024, January 3). *EFFECTS OF ETHANOL EXTRACTS OF EUPHORBIA HIRTA HERB ON SOME OXIDATIVE AND BIOCHEMICAL PARAMETERS IN ALLOXAN-INDUCED DIABETIC RATS*. https://freeresearchpro ject.com.ng/research/effects-of-ethanol-extracts-of-euphorbia-hirta-herb-on-some-oxidative-and-biochemical-parameters-in-alloxan-induced-diabetic-rats/

62 Nahrstedt, A., Schmidt, M., Jäggi, R., Metz, J., & Khayyal, M. T. (2007b). Willow bark extract: The contribution of polyphenols to the overall effect. *Wiener Medizinische Wochenschrift*, 157(13–14), 348–351. https://doi.org/10.1007/s10354-007-0437-3

63 Brekken, R. A., & Sage, E. H. (2001, January 1). *SPARC, a matricellular protein: at the crossroads of cell-matrix communication*. University of Texas Southwestern Medical Center. https://utsouthwestern.pure.elsevier.com/en/publications/sparc-a-matricellular-protein-at-the-crossroads-of-cell-matrix-co

64 Chan, Y. S., Cheng, L., Wu, J., Chan, E., Kwan, Y. W., Lee, S. M., Leung, G. P., Yu, K., & Chan, S. W. (2010). A review of the pharmacological effects of Arctium lappa (burdock). *Inflammopharmacology*, 19(5), 245–254. https://doi.org/10.1007/s10787-010-0062-4

65 Jagdish. (2023, September 12). *10 Profitable Herbal-Based Business Ideas: Low-cost and low-investment manufacturing businesses*. Idea2MakeMoney. https://www.idea2makemoney.com/10-profitable-herbal-based-business-ideas-low-cost-and-low-investment-manufacturing-businesses

66 Admin. (2023b, September 5). The power of natural herbs in healing. *Inoa Juice*. https://inoajuice.com/the-power-of-natural-herbs-in-healing/

67 Plants and Prescriptions. (2022, August 5). *What is herbalism and how does cannabis fit in?* https://plantsandprescriptions.com/2022/08/05/what-is-herbalism-and-how-does-cannabis-fit-in/

68 *Ginkgo Leaf: Ancient Herb, Modern Applications in Herbal Medicine.-Hangzhou Botanical Technology Co., Ltd.* (n.d.-b). https://www.botanic.com.cn/news/ginkgo-leaf--ancient-herb--moder/

69 Kroll. (n.d.-d). *St. John's wort safety in depressed patients: comparison with conventional antidepressants – How to get rid of depression and apathy*. https://elavilnews.com/blog/st-johns-wort-safety-in-depressed-patients-comparison-with-conventional-antidepressants/

70 Stearns, J. (2023b, September 15). *Does taking curcumin for inflammation really*

work? Health Irony | Let's Get Your Longevity to the Next Level! https://www.healthirony.com/curcumin-for-inflammation/

71 *Mulberry Leaf Extract Manufacturer - Herb Green Health.* (n.d.-b). Herb Green Health Biotech Co., Ltd. https://www.herealth.com/products/mulberry-leaf-extract.html

72 *Outdoor Therapy training & Certification Programs | Maryland | CNIT.* (n.d.). CNIT. https://www.natureinformedtherapy.com/nit-training-level1

73 Reed, B. (2023b, December 17). At-Home pain management tips you need to know. *Incrediwear Holdings, Inc.* https://incrediwear.com/blogs/news/at-home-pain-management

74 Maryellen. (2018b, December 19). *FDA warns Kratom products may contain heavy metals | Recall report.* Recall Report. https://www.recallreport.org/2018/12/fda-warns-kratom-products-may-contain-heavy-metals/

75 *Jaundice treatment the natural way with herbal remedies |.* (2017b, March 2). |. http://www.marriageenjoy.com/herbal-remedies-for-jaundice-treatment.html

76 *Silver Needle Tea organic.* (n.d.). Todicamp Store. https://www.todicamp.com/products/organic-silver-needle-tea

77 Lopez, S. (2023b, June 22). What toxins are released after massage? Discover the surprising answer - Phytomer Spa Etoile. *Phytomer Spa Etoile.* https://phytomerspaetoile.com/what-toxins-are-released-after-massage-discover-the-surprising-answer/

78 Healthwave. (2023, September 14). *Alflorex 30 capsules | HealthWave Ireland.* https://healthwave.ie/shop/supplements/alflorex-30-capsules/

79 Sebring, P. L., & Sebring, P. L. (2023b, February 22). How can probiotics benefit you? *Prime Women | An Online Magazine - Redefining the over 50 woman.* https://primewomen.com/wellness/probiotics-for-women/

80 De Beausset Aparicio, S. (2022b, September 18). *Herbal Bitters Review – Is it Effective?* Brain Reference. https://brainreference.com/herbal-bitters-review/

81 *The safety considerations and potential contraindications when using Milkvetch Root.-Hangzhou Botanical Technology Co., Ltd.* (n.d.-b). https://www.botanic.com.cn/news/the-safety-considerations-and-po/

82 Francis, E. A., Teng, L. H., Hadrick, K., & Heinrich, V. (2020b). Density of immobilized antibodies modulates neutrophil biophysical behavior and calcium dynamics during phagocytic spreading. *Biophysical Journal, 118*(3), 605a. https://doi.org/10.1016/j.bpj.2019.11.3269

83 *Healthy Living: Unlocking the 21 secrets of healthy lifestyle.* (n.d.-b). Clinicme. http://www.clinicme.com/2023/08/unlocking-healthy-living-secrets.html

84 Kelly, P., Williamson, C., Niven, A., Hunter, R. F., Mutrie, N., & Richards, J. (2018b). Walking on sunshine: scoping review of the evidence for walking and

mental health. *British Journal of Sports Medicine, 52*(12), 800–806. https://doi.org/ 10.1136/bjsports-2017-098827

85 Energy Healing LLC. (2024b, March 25). *Unseen Connections: Distance Healing with Intention.* Energy Healing. https://energyhealing.pro/distance-healing/

86 *Burdock.* (n.d.). Mount Sinai Health System. https://www.mountsinai.org/health-library/herb/burdock#:~

87 Nutr J. 2014; 13: 20.

Published online 2014 Mar 19. doi: 10.1186/1475-2891-13-20

88 Plants (Basel). 2022 Mar; 11(6): 740.

Published online 2022 Mar 10. doi: 10.3390/plants11060740

89 Vanaspatiteam. (2023, April 17). *Herbal Spotlight: Passionflower.* Vana Tisanes. https://vanatisanes.com/2018/10/30/passionflower/

Made in the USA
Las Vegas, NV
03 December 2024

13236668R00094